The Feldenkrais Method

Power of Self-Transformation

The Feldenkrais Method

Power of Self-Transformation

Abraham Mansbach, Ph.D.

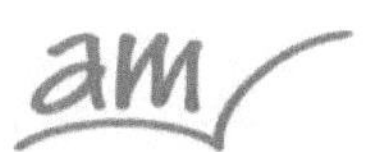

This publication is designed to provide accurate and authoritative information concerning the subject matter covered. The advice and strategies contained herein may not be suitable for every reader. You should consult with a professional when appropriate. Any application of the material set forth in the following pages is at the readers' discretion and their sole responsibility.

Book Cover and Aesthetics by Susanne Kunjappu-Jellinek

Library of Congress Cataloging-in-Publication Data

Mansbach, Abraham, 1949–
    The Feldenkrais Method: Power of Self-Transformation

Includes bibliographical references and index.
ISBN-13: 978-965-598-339-5

1. Feldenkrais Method, 2. Self-Image, 3. Somatics, 4. Kinesthetics, 5. Body Image,
6. Neuroplasticity, 7. Motor development, 8. Psychophysiology. 9. Self-healing,
10. Alternative Therapies.

To Anna and Roie

CONTENTS

Part One: TOWARDS A NEW AND TRUE SELF

Page 2 (facsimile) of Moshe Feldenkrais's manuscript of:

Body and Mature Behavior: A Study of Anxiety, Sex, Gravitation, and Learning

Page 3 (facsimile) of Moshe Feldenkrais's manuscript of:

Body and Mature Behavior: A Study of Anxiety, Sex, Gravitation, and Learning

1. Introduction	1
2. Is the Mental Picture that We Have of Ourselves Accurate?	10
How important is the self-image?	12
What can we learn from the octopus	12
Self-image today	13
How is the self-image formed?	16
Becoming aware of the self-image – The Lessons	18
Perfecting the self-image	23
3. "Why Do We Do Such Strange Movements?"	25
The body has a history	27
The body has a memory	29
What science says about the embodied memory	32
Chronic pain	32
Phantom limb	33
Functional Integration and the body-image:	
Where do you start an FI? How do you do it?	36

Part Two: SELF-CHANGE: THEORY AND PRACTICE

4. The Principles for Self-Transformation 43

5. Reproducing the Motor Development Chain 47

   The Lessons 49

   Balancing and rolling 49

   Rolling to sit 53

   Crawling 56

   Standing to walk 63

6. Reflexes as Archives 68

   The Lessons 69

   Asymmetrical tonic neck reflex 71

   Tonic labyrinthine reflex 76

   Symmetrical tonic neck reflex 79

   Moro reflex 81

7. Habits and Their Renewal: Doing the Same Action Differently 84

   Non-habitual movements – The Lessons 87

   Non-habitual standing 88

   Non-habitual walking 90

8. How Do We Know When a Movement Has Been Mastered? 93

   Doing them Backward – The Lessons 94

   Sitting to lying 94

   Sitting to rolling 95

   Crawling to sitting 96

   Standing to sitting 96

   Walking and standing 97

9. Transformation as Transference 99

Part Three: SENSING THE BODY FROM WITHIN

10. Body Meditation	105
The Lessons	106
Scanning	106
Breathing	108
Bowing–Praying	110
11. Imagination	115
Imagining – The Lessons	119

Part Four: THE SCIENCE OF SELF-TRANSFORMATION

Overture	125
Sensorial Consciousness	127
Brain Plasticity	132
Concern for Oneself and for Others	138
Acknowledgments	141
About the Author	143
Index of Awareness Through Movement (ATM) Lessons	145
Collection of 22 Lessons	151
Index of Names and Terms	153
Selected Bibliography	156

Key to the Feldenkrais Method Lessons

AM   Amherst, 1981–82 Feldenkrais Professional Training

ATM   *Awareness Through Movement: Easy-to-do Health Exercises to Improve Your Posture, Vision, Imagination, and Personal Awareness* (Book)

AY   Alexander Yanai Collection

E   Esalen 1972 Workshop (Recordings)

Es   Esalen 1972 Workshop (Stransky Notes)

PART ONE

TOWARDS A NEW AND TRUE SELF

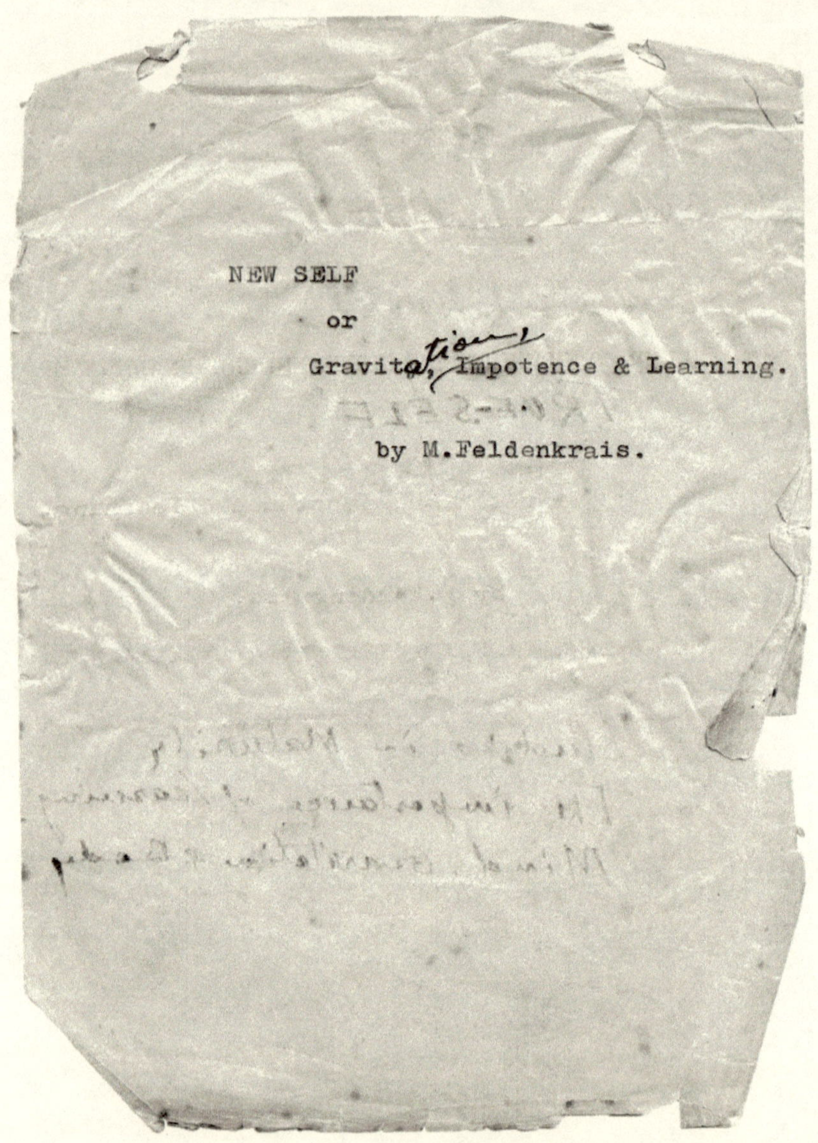

Page 2 of Moshe Feldenkrais's manuscript of:

Body and Mature Behavior: A Study of Anxiety, Sex, Gravitation, and Learning

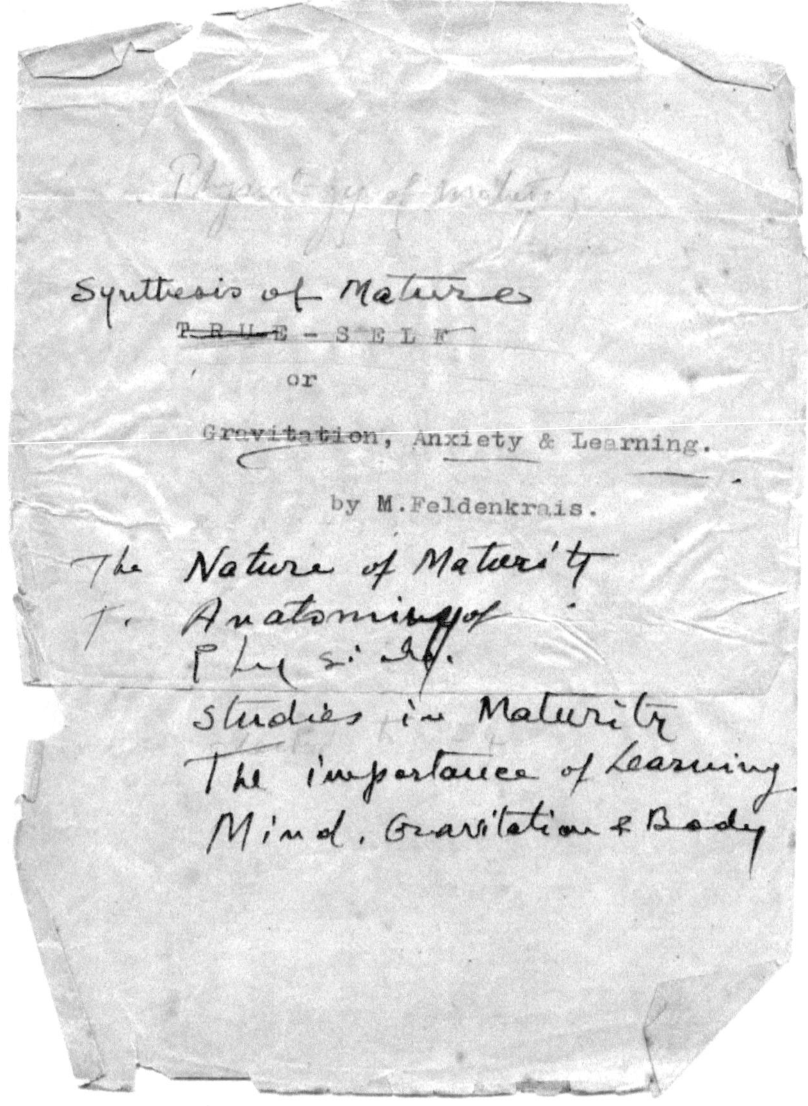

Page 3 of Moshe Feldenkrais's manuscript of:

Body and Mature Behavior: A Study of Anxiety, Sex, Gravitation, and Learning

1

Introduction

Moshe Feldenkrais deleted two titles before the first book he wrote on his method was published as *Body and Mature Behavior: A Study of Anxiety, Sex, Gravitation, and Learning* (1949). The first title was *New Self*, the second *True Self*.[i]

So it is clear that Feldenkrais intended his method to be transformational: a practice that can change individuals by facilitating a richer—more upright, more aware—experience of themselves, in such a way that a new and true self can materialize.

Indeed, one of the things that drew my attention during the four years of my training in the method was the changes that most of the participants were going through. You could perceive gradual changes in their gestures, in the movements of their bodies, and in their ways of interacting with each other. At the end of the training, all of us were

---

[i] I wish to thank the archive of the International Feldenkrais Federation (IFF) for their kind permission to reproduce two pages of the original manuscript of *Body and Mature Behavior: A Study of Anxiety, Sex, Gravitation, and Learning*, by Moshe Feldenkrais.

different from when it started. We all had a different body schema. I imagine that this happens to all those who practice the method, though perhaps with dissimilarities in intensity or pace, or just differently.

That the Feldenkrais Method can change those who practice it is a message that figures prominently throughout Feldenkrais's teaching and writings. The message is corroborated by our own experiences, whether as students of the method or practitioners who perceive the changes in those who take part in Functional Integration (FI) and Awareness through Movement (ATM) lessons.[i]

The idea of a somatic practice of self-change intrigues me further as a philosopher who has been exploring the theme of identity and selfhood, trying to answer questions such as: How do we become who we are? What are the energies and dynamism that shape us and give us an identity? Are we autonomous and free to forge ourselves at will? Or is our existential status like that of marionettes who are made and moved by forces "out there," beyond our will and control? Or are these rather two poles of a spectrum? And if so, how can we move along it?

---

[i] The Feldenkrais Method is taught through two modalities. Awareness through Movement (ATM) lessons are a series of guided movement sequences, in which the participant is verbally led by the practitioner. The lessons are similar to those of tai chi, qigong, and gentle yoga in the softness and mindfulness with which the movements are carried out. A class may last somewhere between 35 and 50 minutes. The participants may walk, stand, or lie on the floor in one or more of a variety of comfortable positions. The second modality, Functional Integration (FI), is a one-to-one encounter where the practitioner uses her/his hands to perform smooth, noninvasive, and non-painful movements with the skeleton and the musculature of the learner. This precise manual contact mirrors the student's organization of their body configuration. The idea is to join with the student's body organization and movements, so as to bring the student's awareness to them (chapters 3, and 9).

During this inquiry, *the body* has drawn many of my efforts, as I have tried to elucidate its significance in the equation: How is the body related to the self? In this regard, I have studied how the human body is shaped by culture, by the experiences of early childhood, by the practices that we engage in, by the gaze of other people on us, by the images projected by the electronic and social media, by the spaces that we inhabit, as well as how brain processes play out in the theater of the body. Practicing the Feldenkrais Method and exploring its general principles have added a new facet to this inquiry.

A common view regarding the self or self-image is that it consists of the behavioral, mental, emotional, or spiritual aspects of the person. The Feldenkrais Method is informed by a different view, which says that the key to the self-image is in the body and its movements.

The idea supporting this view is the unity between the self and the body, not as a unity of two different things, but rather as one thing. In Feldenkrais's words, "the self or self-image is the body-image."[i] In his lessons, lectures, and writings, Feldenkrais uses the notions of self, self-image, and body-image interchangeably. I will follow his usage here.

Certainly, Feldenkrais was not the first to affirm such unity, and he won't be the last. He was also not the first to regard the body, its movements, and its practices as constitutive and defining of a person's identity.[ii] However, what is distinctive is that by modeling a series of somatic practices, a method, he made such an idea tangible.

---

[i] AY 024: "The Body Image, a Lecture" – (Reels 2/4/1 and 2/4/3).

[ii] On "body culture," a theme trending in the 1920s in Europe that influenced Feldenkrais, see Thomas Kampe's "Dancing the Soma-Ecstatic: Feldenkrais and the Modernist Body," in Scholl 2021, chap.1.

Indeed, the Feldenkrais Method is built on this idea of embodied oneness, and the most amazing fact is that by practicing the method, we can experience this integral unity. To be sure, the Feldenkrais Method generates changes in the organization of the body's movements, in its flexibility, and in acquiring comfortable bodily organization for sitting, standing, walking, and diverse activities of everyday life, such as lifting heavy objects. Given that there is no movement without sensation, no sensation without feeling, and no feeling without thought, with continued practice the changes become functional modifications that resonate with the person's affects, sensations, emotions, and thoughts. The unity that the Feldenkrais Method refers to is the integration of all the layers of sensorimotor experience.

The Feldenkrais Method reorganizes the body's configuration by integrating anew its different parts and their articulations, and with this their wiring in the nervous system and brain, as well as the self-image, are enlivened. To be sure, bodily pains and tensions that are the result of inadequate carriage and poorly organized movements can be eased in a series of ATM or FI lessons. Long-lasting modifications of the body movements and the sensorial layer, and the renewal of the self-image, however, are the result of a regular and suitable practice, in which small and micro-changes accumulate over time, and of a concurrent process of somatic awareness.

The notion that changes in the body can generate changes in the self or self-image might seem trivial. Nowadays, people change their bodies through different means and ways and become somehow different. Dietary regimes, bodybuilding, extreme tattooing, plastic surgery, gender affirmation surgery, practices of self-harm or self-mutilation, and others modify the body and might transform the self-image as well.

The Feldenkrais method differs from all of them in many ways; noticeable is the pace of the changes and the kinesthetic awareness required for a self-modification to take effect. To be sure, the method belongs to a distinct category of somatic practices, among which we find a group of Chinese martial arts known as "internal arts," such as qigong and tai chi, as well as Japanese aikido, the Alexander Technique, and some forms of yoga.[i] While these are all different practices with different cultural roots, they all have a family resemblance.

Properties that characterize this family of practices are the fusion of body and mind, control of movements and breathing, developing a more optimal posture and flexibility, increasing the range of mobility, generating internal energy, mindfulness, and kinesthetic awareness, among others. While the distribution and the emphasis of these features are not uniform among the different techniques, they all share this: they are self-healing practices.

The self-healing power of the Feldenkrais Method manifests at various levels and is to be understood in a wide sense. There is a long list of evidence-based research on a range of ailments for which the method has been effective, relieving chronic conditions and pain and improving the movement of individuals with many kinds of bodily impairments.[ii] The Feldenkrais Method has been used, as well, to

---

[i] Chinese martial arts are classified as of two kinds: the external arts and the internal arts. The external arts focus their training methods on developing muscular strength, speed, and athletic prowess. The internal arts stress relaxation, mind-intention, balance to actuate vital force, which does not rely on athleticism and muscular strength.

[ii] Some of the studies published in double-blind peer-reviewed scientific journals and books are in rehabilitation, physical medicine, eating disorders, anxiety, gerontology, and chronic pain. Under the words "Feldenkrais Therapy,"

positively assist people with central nervous system conditions such as multiple sclerosis, cerebral palsy, stroke, and Parkinson's.[i] There are also innumerable undocumented cases of practitioners, patients, and students who have experienced the healing benefits of the method. It is important to emphasize, though, that the Feldenkrais Method is not intended exclusively for people who suffer from some condition, mobility deficiency, or impairment. Self-healing is indeed part and parcel of the power of self-change; the method, however, goes well beyond physical health. The method is aimed and apt for anyone who aspires to feel better in and with themselves by being more in sync with their embodied self, so that a truer self can emerge.

Being more in sync means fine-tuning movements, actions, feelings, and behavior to refine the self-image. Certainly, a regular practice of the method can reintegrate the diverse layers of the sensorimotor apparatus. This has many benefits: by distributing the energy used in our movements more efficiently, it reinforces self-esteem and heightens assertiveness and confidence, which in the end renders the handling of everyday life and the choosing of courses of action smoother, increasing the ease and joy of living. As a thread that weaves physical, emotional, and mental well-being, a Feldenkrais practice makes individuals the architects and keepers of their self-image.

The question that intrigues me most is: How does the Feldenkrais Method generate such changes? What are the principles of the method, and how are they staged in practice? This is indeed a challenging task, as Feldenkrais himself acknowledged in the preface to

---

the web search engine Google Scholar has more than 8000 entries (accessed January 10, 2022).

[i] A search in Google Scholar on the words "Feldenkrais" and "Parkinson" has more than 1200 entries of professional publications (January 10, 2022).

The Elusive Obvious: "I have tried to write what is necessary for you to understand *how* my techniques work ... we really only know how." [emphasis in original][i]

Putting the onus on the practice of the method, rather than on the theory that sustains it, highlights the complexity of making explicit the principles of such a multilayered method. Moreover, Feldenkrais did not consider theory and practice as two different things. He asserted that "my theory is thought in such an organic way that theory and practice, action and thinking, feeling and senses, are all one."[ii]

To face the challenge, in this book I offer a theory of the power of self-change of the Feldenkrais Method and, at the same time, the practice of the theory, by bringing exemplary lessons selected from the large corpus that Feldenkrais left us, staging the principles of the process of transformation.

The Feldenkrais Method is a very rich practice that can be examined through different perspectives, and the lessons can be categorized according to different themes. One such organizing principle can be the initial position, such as standing lessons, lying on the back, or chair lessons. Another grouping can be according to the parts of the body that are at the center of the lessons, such as head and neck, ribs, or pelvis. Balance can also be a theme under which lessons are pieced together. These perspectives are all beneficial, with enormous value for learning, practicing, and enjoying the benefits of the method. The lessons chosen in this book show how self-transformation is achieved through the Feldenkrais Method, which, I believe, is the theme that goes to the heart of the method. The ultimate aim is to give a cohesive

---

[i] *The Elusive Obvious*, p.1.

[ii] AM 1 – Week 3 – June 23 AM1: "Lying on stomach (continued)."

picture of the power of change of the Feldenkrais Method, while at the same time offering a guide to practice, cultivate the method, and refine the body-self-image.

The trajectory is as follows: The book has four parts divided into chapters. The first three parts examine Feldenkrais Method lessons that address the themes in question, showing how these themes are activated and staged in the method.

The first theme is the self-body image: how it takes form, and its importance to the well-being of every person. I analyze several lessons that enhance somatic awareness of the self-image by using various sensorial channels such as imagination, scanning, and movement resonance, which is activated when the movement of parts of the body that are sensed reverberates through those that are not. Attention then turns to the body's memory and history as the sources that orchestrate the dynamics of the body's movements.

The second theme is the theory and the practice of self-transformation. Here, I describe the three-pronged strategy of the method to enhance sensorial-kinesthetic awareness of somatic patterns and memories. The first is to revise the blueprint of the primary movements, which is done by reproducing the experience of learning how to roll, sit up, crawl, stand up, and walk. The second is to replicate and revitalize prenatal and early-life reflexes, which are the building blocks of sensorimotor development. The third consists in resetting and renewing habitual movements. To finalize, I present what it means to master a movement, and share a pair of lessons that epitomize how transformation is attained.

In the third part, I explore imagination and body-meditation, which are two channels that the method uses to sense the body from within, thereby awakening somatic awareness and accessing the sensorial consciousness. I examine lessons that perform three modes of body meditation: scanning, breathing, and bowing-praying.

The last part of the book outlines the scientific basis of the power of transformation and offers a glance at the method from the perspective of the brain and neuroscience. Here, I look at two areas where the method meets neuroscience: the interaction between consciousness and nonconscious processes, and neuroplasticity, which embodies our ability to change neural networks in the brain. Lastly, I place the method at the crossroads of ethics and neuroscience, as an art of self-fashioning in which agency blends with responsibility for oneself and others, enacting the needs and drives of the organism and the brain while promoting the growth and integration of the embodied self.

2

Is the Mental Picture that We Have of Ourselves Accurate?

Self-image is the mental picture that human beings have of themselves. The image is formed by a variety of aspects, but essentially by the physical characteristics that can be objectively described, such as height, shape, weight, hair color, as well as by what every person has absorbed, adopted, and internalized from their life experiences, including social and cultural ideas, emotional attitudes, and values.

By and large, people believe that the mental picture they have of themselves accurately reflects how they objectively are. But even at the physical level, this assumption is, in most cases, inaccurate. Feldenkrais demonstrates this on different occasions through simple tests. Here is one of them that you can try on your own, and with family, friends, and students: "Close your eyes, and using the index fingers of each hand, without touching each other or any other part of the body, try to indicate the length of your mouth." [i] When you finish, open your eyes and compare.

Usually, the measurement does not correspond to the actual length of the mouth and can be several times too large or too small. Given that we look at our mouth in the mirror three or four times a day on average, the results are surprising. The test can also be made with other parts of the body, such as the thickness of the chest or the thigh, with similar results.[ii]

The inaccuracy of how we experience ourselves is due to the complexity of the self-image, which is configured by diverse factors. These include the organization and the movements of the body, the layers of human experience that accompany the movements, such as sensations, emotions, and thoughts, as well as their wiring in the nervous system and brain. In Feldenkrais's words:

> Self-image … is a body image; namely, it is the shape and relationship of the bodily parts, which means the spatial and temporal relationships, as well as the kinesthetic feelings. Included with these are feelings and emotions and one's thoughts. All of these form an integrated whole.[iii]

Before I give a more detailed account of how the self-image takes form, and introduce lessons that facilitate having a more precise image of ourselves, let me first answer the question: Why is it important to have a

---

[i] "Image, Movement, and Actor," p. 115. See also *Embodied Wisdom*, p. 9.

[ii] See *Awareness Through Movement*, p. 22, and AY 026: "Pearls and Eyes" – (Reel 2/4/5).

[iii] *Embodied Wisdom*, p. 3.

more rather than less accurate self-image? What are the benefits of having the self-image "in sync," and the inconveniences and even hazards of being out of sync? We can get a clue from the octopus.

How important is the self-image?

What can we learn from the octopus?
There are many different kinds of changes in appearance and body-image that we witness in nature. One of them, and most amazing, is that of the octopus. Octopuses transform their body in such a way that they can mimic the color, texture, shape, size, and relations of the different parts of their immediate environment, whether it is a coral reef, a rocky surface, an aquatic plant, a sponge garden, or seaweed.

Do octopuses have a body-image in their central brain that enables them to do such sophisticated maneuvers? Are they aware of how they look, and do they, consequently, know how to transform themselves to emulate their environment? Is this mechanism a form of self-consciousness?

An answer to these interesting questions goes beyond the limits of this book; it will suffice to say here that whether it lies in the octopuses' central brain, in the nerve fibers of their arms, or in the distinctive configuration of their nervous system, the fact is that such knowledge is part of their organism. The knowledge resides in the nervous system, and it encompasses sensation and action. The octopus senses its environment, it senses danger when there is a predator in the area and appetizing opportunity when there is prey, and action is generated accordingly.[i]

---

[i] See Godfrey-Smith 2017, on the mental complexity of invertebrate animals such as the octopus.

We can imagine that if an octopus's organism were to lose or "forget" such knowledge after suffering some damage to the nervous system, so that the mimicking of the environment and camouflaging went wrong, it could not avoid its predators, and would not survive long. For human beings, it is only in very extreme cases that an inaccurate or distorted self-image can have fatal consequences. However, misrepresentations of the body-image, whether large or small, resonate with the behavior and the feelings of the person and can affect physical and emotional well-being. This can obstruct self-realization, satisfaction, social interaction, and accomplishment. To be sure, for human beings their self-image is of great importance in ways that it is not for octopuses.

Self-image today

We live in times when self-image has become of utmost importance. People care about the way they look, and the way they feel and think about their looks. While one of the most common stereotypes is that young women are uneasy about their appearance more than any other group of the population, research has shown that self-image is a concern for all ages and genders.[i] There are transition points in people's lives, such as puberty, pregnancy, parenthood, menopause, when the

---

[i] We should notice that there is a confirmation bias in the research on body-image that feeds the stereotype that young women are more concerned about their appearance than any other group of the population — but that is because social scientists have done the overwhelming majority of their body-image research on young women. For research showing that self-image is a concern for all ages and genders, see Mental Health Foundation 2019. https://www.metalhealth.org.uk/sites/deault/files/DqVNbWRVvpAPQzw.pdf, accessed August 15, 2021.

hair starts turning silver, reaching age sixty-five, mourning, or retirement, when concern about the self-image intensifies and creates tensions, due to the need to adjust to expected as well as unexpected changes.

Fine-tuning the self-image to the changes in life can be a not-so-easy task in and of itself. The difficulties are exacerbated in today's reality of celebrity culture and social media, where "body image" is constantly under discussion and scrutiny, and the way we perceive ourselves passes through the gaze of other people on us, through the mirroring effect of the internet, or in a liked or disliked photograph or video circulating on social media.

A large number of studies have shown that having concerns about how one looks and having a poor self-image, can affect one with different grades of intensity in one's physical, emotional, social, and mental realms. It can be a risk factor affecting health and generating psychosomatic pains, as well as a range of unhealthy feelings and behaviors, such as depression and anxiety. In more extreme cases it can trigger eating disorders, and even self-harm, while mild imprecisions of the self-image can diminish personal qualities and hinder self-realization.[i]

Furthermore, the images projected by the media, both social and commercial, that influence how we feel in and about our bodies, generate patterns that homogenize the individual. To be similar to others

---

[i] An internal study Facebook conducted over three years (2018–2020) found that Instagram makes body-image issues worse for roughly one in three teen girls. In the survey, teens also said that Instagram increased rates of anxiety and depression. See https://www.wsj.com/articles/facebook-knows-instagram-is-toxic-for-teen-girls-company-documents-show-11631620739?mod=article_inline.

has benefits, such as the ease with which individuals integrate into society; however, singularity and uniqueness are in peril, and with their loss, individual capabilities and potentialities can be limited and even thwarted.[i]

By attuning the self-image, the Feldenkrais Method avoids blurring the differences between individuals, overshadowing their identities, and succumbing to the homogenization process prevalent in our societies. The uniqueness of each person is a basic idea in the practice of the method, and a pedagogical and didactic tool of its practitioners. The Feldenkrais Method does not offer a model of how each movement should exactly and unerringly be made. Instructions given in the lessons are not orders to move according to some prototype or in a very precise way, as in gymnastics. When in a lesson the instruction is "to raise a hand" or "to roll the head," what is expected from the participant is to move the limb or part of the body in a specific direction and pace. The idea is that each individual makes the movements in their own way, as the sensorimotor organization and make-up of their body facilitate. This is a *sine qua non* of the method, aiming to foster the uniqueness of every person, and to improve the integration of the body's movements and the awareness of its configuration, thereby nurturing a truer self.

We should notice, however, that having the physical, sensorial, emotional, and cognitive layers of the self-image in full sync is not an easy task; moreover, Feldenkrais asserts that "A complete self-image is an ideal rarely attained."[ii] I should add that the self is a process, not

---

[i] For Feldenkrais's view on the problem of homogenization in society, see AY 303: "A Lecture/Lesson: Self-image Lecture, the Line of a Ball that Rolls" – (Reel 21/1/3).

[ii] *Embodied Wisdom*, p. 9.

an inert thing, and the self-image may change concurrently with the changes that each person undergoes throughout life. Thus, the question is not how to attain perfect synchronization of the different layers of the sensorimotor body schema—which at the moment of its attainment is short-lived—but how the adequacy of the self-image can be improved, in the sense of a gradual bettering which has no limit.[i] The Feldenkrais Method, like other methods of the same family, is a system and collection of practices and lessons pursuing continuous improvement.

How is the self-image formed?

Feldenkrais describes the self-image as formed through a combination of three main sources: heritage, education, and self-education. **Heritage** is" the biological endowment of the individual,"[ii] which corresponds to the human body in all its materiality, including the nervous system, the skeletal system, the internal organs, the muscles, the genetic code, as well as the configuration and functioning of all limbs, parts, and organs of the body.

Education, here, is not limited to the knowledge that can be acquired at an educational institution but is far more comprehensive. The notion refers to culture in general. It encompasses what we, as human beings, learn from the world in which we live and the family we grow up in. It includes the spoken language, the concepts used to understand and describe the surrounding world, acquired values and habits, norms adopted from society and family, and everyday practices such as the way we dress and prepare our food. In short,

---

[i] On self-improvement see *The Potent Self*, ch.11.

[ii] *Awareness Through Movement*, p. 3.

education encompasses everything that is learned, embraced, and appropriated from the human and the natural environments.

It is pertinent to note, in this regard, that Feldenkrais was highly critical of certain important aspects of the social arrangements of his time. He asserts—and this can be applied to our times as well—that "[i]t is hard to deny that the traditional foundations of our social structure need thorough revision. No objective observer, free of prejudice, will argue against the necessity of radical changes."[i] Feldenkrais thought of his method as a practice for personal change, but whether he conceived it or not as a means that might help to revise the social organization is an open question (see Part Four).

The third source is **self-education**. This element is unique and represents what every person does to mold one's self. Its importance cannot be overstated since, of the three sources that constitute the self-image, self-education is the only one that is "in our hands."[ii] We cannot change our biological endowment at will. The cultural legacy that we acquire from our human environment, and the emotional molding from our family and community, is not something that is in the individual's hands to fashion according to his or her interest. It is in the third element, self-education, that we find the "mechanism" for self-molding and self-change.

Self-education develops from the very early stages of life; it is a process through which the individual's characteristics take shape. This process involves the distinctive features of the environment where the person's sensorimotor development takes place; the physical activities that they choose to engage in; the adoption and internalization of

---

[i] *Body and Mature Behavior*, p. 10.

[ii] *Awareness Through Movement*, p. 4.

behavior and practices that are acceptable to others, as well as forms of resistance to and rejection of behavior that the person finds unacceptable, not fitting their felt sense of self. Self-education represents the personal dynamics that foster and give expression to what is unique in every individual. Feldenkrais defines it as an "active force that extends inherited difference into the realm of action,"[i] giving rise to acts or practices through which the uniqueness of each person is nurtured and expressed.

The Feldenkrais Method is a practice of self-education that instructs how to functionally integrate the body movements and the sensorial layers as an active force of self-making, self-sustaining, and self-transformation.

Becoming aware of the self-image – The Lessons

The Feldenkrais Method as a whole aims to enhance somatic awareness of the self-image. There are, however, several lessons that specifically focus on this endeavor. These lessons serve to initiate participants into becoming aware of their self-image configuration and attentive to its features.

The template for the self-image is, basically, composed of five "cardinal lines" representing the large body parts, which are the two arms, two legs, and the spinal column. It is a simple schema that "even a child could identify as a human body…when we add a small circle on the top."[ii] We should notice that the "five cardinal lines" image, though simple, is an important device for heightening and deepening

---

[i] Ibid.

[ii] E 2: "Scanning and General Remarks"

somatic awareness, since these "lines" are the actors in and activators of the body's movements.

Feldenkrais notes that the cardinal lines are the most basic schema of the human being, and, as such, they have a correlate design at the level of the nervous system and the brain. The schema is indeed the "foundation of the human organism" and the skeletal system; it is its cardinal structure.[i]

In the lessons that I have selected, we can see how the figure of five lines, "strings" or "sticks" as they are sometimes called, is constructed, and how from being a simple schema, it further develops, gaining in suppleness, depth, and strength.

The five lines theme appears in several lessons. One that stages it in an inspiring and compelling way is "Scanning." The importance of this lesson for the self-image theme cannot be overemphasized. "Scanning" is the opening lesson of the Esalen workshop that Feldenkrais gave in 1972, which was an important and very meticulously planned encounter.[ii]

> *E 2: Scanning and General Remarks/Es 1: Scanning* [iii]
> In this lesson, the five lines' primary self-image is built
> in the background of scanning all parts of the body, the
> movements of the eyes, the shoulders, the head, the
> legs, and the breathing rhythm.

---

[i] AY 333: "Movement of Opposition" – (Reel 23/1/1).

[ii] The Esalen Workshop lasted for 5–6 weeks, at the end of which the group of 14 participants were accredited to teach the method. All of the participants had some specialty in somatic studies and practice. See David Zemach-Bersin's "Introduction" in *Esalen 1972 Workshop*.

[iii] The titles and the numbers of the Esalen recordings are different from Judith Stransky's Notes. I will quote "E (recordings)/Es (Stransky)."

The image is built in three steps. First, a slow scanning of the parts of the body represented by each line— two legs, two arms, and the spinal column. The scanning is assisted by two imaginary fingers that exert pressure while moving along the spine. In the second step, the image is kept in the back of the mind, during which parts of the body are moved and differentiated from each other, such as the right from the left shoulder, the head from the shoulders, and each shoulder from its opposite hip. In the last step, the five-line figure is retrieved, and compared to the initial image at the opening of the lesson.

The idea in this lesson is that participants go back and forth from the initial awareness of the self-image to the one experienced throughout the different movements. The objective is to assemble the self-image by distinguishing the changes being undergone and the movements generating them. Going back and forth and exploring the variations in the five lines' self-image, is an important didactic tool that is effectively used in many lessons.

AY 337: Knots – (Reel 23/1/5)

In this lesson, the self-image formed by the cardinal lines becomes clearer by tying an imaginary rope around different parts of the body, such as a knee, an elbow, the bridge of the nose, and the hip joints. The knot of the rope travels along and around all the parts, touching and stimulating the feeling of them. The length and direction of the spine, the arms, and the legs are sensorially revitalized through an imaginary push from the sacrum that activates the spine upwards.

AY 338: Primary Image – (Reel 23/2/1)

In this lesson, the stick figure becomes less simple by adding two horizontal lines to the existing five. One is the line of the shoulders, where the two arms are actually connected. The other is the line of the hips, which connects the legs. The two added lines are in charge of the gyrating-turning movement of the body, and in the lesson they are activated from both a sitting and a lying position, by a slight rolling to the sides.

In essence, this lesson gives a geometrical perspective to the self-image. The shoulders and the hip joints become points of their respective lines. The rolling movements are made without altering the distances between the points and the lines, thereby maintaining the symmetry of the plane formed by four points, the two of the shoulders and the two of the hips. The attention is neither in the body itself nor in the shapes of the hip and shoulder bones, but rather in the abstract figure formed by lines and points. Length and direction, rather than volume, form the ethereal, insubstantial image.

AY 122.2: Repose (this is your skeleton) – (Reel 9/3/2)[i]

In this lesson, the self-image is enlivened via movement transmitted by and through the body. With the arms extended above the head, a diagonal scanning travels through the small bones and the main articulations of the body. The scanning goes from the bones of the fingers of the hand toward the toes of the opposite foot, in slow, light movements of the ankles, the knees, and the shoulders. Essentially, this lesson enhances perception of the micro-dimension of the lines of the self-image, as well as of the movement and its transmission throughout the body. The lesson further refines the self-image by underlining the diagonal lines of the body.

AY 339: Simpler – (Reel 23/2/2)

This lesson bridges between refining awareness of the cardinal lines and perfecting the self-image. At the basis of the refinement is the schema of the body formed by the seven lines constructed as an abstract figure, and designed by the length and direction of the lines and the width of the body, rather than by the volume and size of the bones. Awareness of the cardinal structure is ensured by sensing, imagining, or visualizing the full length of the spine, the distances between the five vertical lines, and the places where arms and legs connect, in the shoulders and the hips, with the spine.

---

[i] This lesson is not included in the Alexander Yanai Collections.

Concerning the process of perfecting the self-image, this lesson focuses on sections of the spine and the back that are usually not sensed and integrates them into the movements of the whole spine, by pinpointing the places in the back where a movement resonates.

Perfecting the self-image

There are parts of the body where, even when they are active, sensation is fuzzy or nonexistent. To refine and perfect the self-image, these parts have to be integrated into the awareness schema. The way the Feldenkrais Method does that is by bracketing together those parts of the body with other parts that are sensorially present. In the previous lesson (AY 339), the movement of parts of the spine that are sensed resonates with those that are not. In the next three lessons, we can see how scanning and imagination—two themes examined in chapters 10 and 11—blend to expand awareness of areas of the body that are sensorially vague or muted, thereby perfecting the self-image.

E 46: Imagination and Action to Complete the Back Self-Image [i]
ATM Lesson 11: Becoming Aware of Parts of Which We are not Conscious
AY 303: Self-image Lecture, the Line of a Ball that Rolls – (Reel 21/1/3)

The central motif of these similar lessons is to prompt awareness of parts of the back of the body that are not usually sensed. The means for doing this is by scanning the body, helped by the imagination.

---

[i] This lesson is not included in Judith Stransky's Notes.

Lying face down, a slow scanning starts from one heel and travels upward all the way through the back and all its different parts, then on in the direction of the opposite extended hand. Imagining, thinking, and sensing together smooth the scanning. An imaginary finger initiates the scanning by pressing the heel; then an imaginary small iron ball continues by rolling from the heel upward all through the back of the body. An imaginary lifting of the leg rolls the ball in the direction of the hand, and an imaginary lifting of the hand rolls the ball back in the direction of the heel. The ball rolls through the different parts of the back of the body, following the path of least resistance. In E 46, scanning marks the diagonal lines of the body, emphasizing the lines of pressure that link each hand to its opposite foot, thereby refining the cardinal schema.

We saw in these lessons how awareness of the template that composes the self-image is enhanced through three sensorial channels: imagination, scanning, and movement resonance. The next step is to look at what orchestrates the body movements.

3

"Why Do We Do Such Strange Movements?"

In the lesson "The Body Image, a Lecture," speaking about his method, Feldenkrais asks: "Why do we do what we do?" and "Why do we do such strange movements?" [i] To answer, he borrows from the tri-dimensional schema of Paul Schilder, the scientist who introduced the terms "body-image" and "body schema" in 1935.[ii]

One dimension is the external and observable features of the body, such as height, size, hair, skin color, complexion, facial features, and the overall build of the body. The second is the representation of the

---

[i] AY 024 – (Reels 2/4/1 and 2/4/3).

[ii] Schilder's ideas on psychology were a source of inspiration for Feldenkrais. Schilder explored the role of changes in body image in different emotional and mental pathologies, concerning feelings of depersonalization. His concept of body image encompasses modes of spatiality, movement, perception, emotion, personality, sexuality, and social functioning (Schilder 1935). On the influence of Schilder on Feldenkrais, see Reese 2015, chaps. 2, 4, and 6.

body parts and their movements in the brain, specifically in the motor cortex.[i] The third dimension is what each of us feels when we say "I," "my voice," "my eyes," "my hands," "my feelings, or "my thoughts." [ii]

What Feldenkrais offers with his method, and its "strange movements," is a set of practices that aims to functionally integrate the three different tiers that configure the self-image (the physical, the sensory-psychological, and the neurological) and to fuse them all into an organic whole, as one.

The integration is informed by two main principles: one, the body has a history; and two, the body has a memory. Having a history means that the body, its movements, and its posture have been and continue to be shaped throughout time by the ample gamut of interactions with the human, the cultural, and the natural environments. Having a memory refers to the fact that the schema and configuration of the body, as it is shaped through time, is imprinted in the nervous

---

[i] The representation of the body in the motor cortex is known as the *homunculus*. The term describes a suppositional map in the brain of input from sensory neurons or output to motor neurons corresponding to parts of the body. The neuroscientist Antonio Damasio rejects the idea of the homunculus as it was originally represented: as an all-knower. For him, "a homunculus-like knower, endowed with full knowledge and located in a single and circumscribed part of the brain, makes no sense physiologically." (Damasio 1999, p.190) For Feldenkrais's opinion on the homunculus, see AY 303: "A Lecture/Lesson: Self-image Lecture, the Line of a Ball that Rolls" – (Reel 21/1/3).

[ii] It should be noted that what neuroscience has to say today on the interaction of these three dimensions in shaping the self, or I, and on the areas, states, or activities of the brain that correlate with "I" and "my," is different. For Damasio, for instance, it is the continuity of the body itself, its invariance, and its representation in the brain that anchors the mental self, the I. See Damasio 2003. For more on Damasio and Feldenkrais, see Part Four below.

system, a material memory of sorts that is active in the organism, in the body, and in its skeletal construct.

The body has a history

The way our body is structured and designed has been determined by two specific sources. One is the personal body-history, the ontogenetic; the other is the history of the body as it developed in the human species — the phylogenetic.

Regarding the skeletal system, this bony structure has basic properties that all human beings share, which include the relative size of each bone in comparison to the others, its shape, its position, weight, and strength, as well as the attached muscles, nerves, and ligaments, which regulate the dynamic relations at play in the movements of the assemblage.

The pattern of motor development is, in general, shared by all human beings as well. Indeed, every human being has the potential to walk at approximately twelve months of age, to ride a bicycle at five years old, to learn to rollerblade and skateboard from an early age too, to learn how to play a complex game like football, baseball, or cricket — even to learn to walk on a tightrope.

All of these activities, and many others that people can perform, involve knowing the relative positions of the parts of one's body both in movement and in stillness. This is possible due to the sense of balance that human beings have. This proprioceptive sense is the outcome of an evolutionary process over millions of years, in which organisms in general, and the human species in particular, have gone through adjustment of their movements to the force of gravity.[i] There are also other senses that aim to achieve effective integration of the body in, and with, its environment, such as thermoception, by which an organism perceives temperatures, and nociception, the sensation of pain. These senses are part of the apparatus of life management designed to preserve and enrich life. It is information inscribed in the organism of every human being, and of other living beings as well, that serves as an unbeatable adaptive force and functionality.

In addition to what all human beings share of their body's development and its dynamics are the differences between individuals informed by the uniqueness of their body-history. This history comprises many factors, such as the genetic code, the conditions of birth, the way the newborn is carried by his or her caretaker; the learning processes of rolling, crawling, sitting, standing, and walking; the way stimuli and constraints intervening in those processes are handled by the infant, as well as the affects and feelings prompted during development. There are also modifications of body posture and movements that are the result of the work that people do, of physical education and fitness, of the physical distresses and traumas suffered through injuries, ailments, and genetic or accidentally caused disabilities. Furthermore, the personal body-history is also the outcome of adjustments to conditions of life, such as climate, environmental conditions, and diet.

Changes in the personal body-history usually come in tandem with changes in the self-image. From the day that we were born, our

---

[i] Proprioception has also been identified in other vertebrate animals and in some invertebrates, such as arthropods. More recently, proprioception has also been described in flowering land plants. On the challenge that bipedalism faces vis à vis the force of gravity and the relation to the spine, see Le Huec et al. 2011.

size, weight, and volume have significantly changed. The representation of the body in the brain has adjusted accordingly. Motor developments, games and sports that we played, physical work, skilled and semi-skilled activities, habits, all that we have learned, read, and written, norms and values, have changed our bodies, our feelings, and our mental capacities. These practices plow new paths in our brain and connections between our neurons. When we say "my thoughts," "my feelings," "my voice," or "my hands," the "I" to which these expressions refer has changed throughout time as well.

The double-axis formation of the history of the body, which combines the personal dimension with what is inherent in every human organism and skeletal system, orchestrates the dynamics of the body's movements. To be sure, this is a guiding principle of the Feldenkrais Method as well as a pedagogical tool for its teaching and its practice. The method operates at both the phylogenetic and the ontogenetic level of the history of the body, to restore functionality to the skeletal system, its organization, its movements and posture.

The body has a memory

Memory is generally referred to as a faculty of the mind that stores and accesses information. It is the mental capacity of retaining and reviving facts, events, and impressions, as well as recalling or recognizing previous experiences. In the present context, I am referring to a different type of memory, a memory of the organism, a material-sensorial memory. This memory stores the information from the two sources of the history of the body. One is the information owned by virtue of being a member of the human species, and embedded and kept within the organism. The other source is the sensorimotor memories of personal events that the individual has gone through, whether in the preverbal stage as a newborn and infant, in very early childhood, or at some moment in the person's life.

The knowledge that the human body carries by nature, such as the primitive reflexes that form the basis of motor development, are features encoded genetically, inherited from the forebears, and preserved by every person for further transmission. Instincts are also a case in point. While it is true that we do not climb a tree when we sense danger close by, as some of our ancestors probably did, we too react in flight or fight mode in the face of danger. These actions are not taken after a thoughtful decision; they are rapid reactions of the nervous system, specifically of the sympathetic system. It is a survival reaction encrypted and preserved in the nervous system of every member of the human species (and other living beings), and adapted to the different environments and forms of life that human beings face. It is a material knowledge of sorts, a knowledge of the body by the body itself, without our being consciously aware of it. A nonconscious form of knowledge.

Among sensorimotor personal memories we can count, for instance, the specific way in which each person experienced his or her motor development—the obstacles, or lack of them, in the process of going from rolling to sitting, to crawling and standing. Habitual body patterns and gestures acquired by nonconscious mimicry within the family, or the community fall in this category as well. Included also are bodily adjustments to the work that each one does and to the practices of everyday life.

Sensory memories from the two sources are not accessed through cognitive recollection or by calling them to mind; nonetheless, they are not forgotten. Furthermore, this information is available and can surface in our behavior as acts and as feelings, often triggered by experiences patterned similarly to the original ones. In the words of the neuroscientist Antonio Damasio:

> All of our memories, inherited from evolution and available at birth or acquired through learning thereafter… exist in our brains in dispositional form, waiting to become explicit images or actions.[i]

Needless to say, the information stored in the body's memory is highly important to the self-image. It is, certainly, one of its major constituents, as Feldenkrais reminds us: "It is impossible to forget the past without forgetting oneself at the same time." Forgetting oneself makes it difficult, if not impossible, to attune the self-image. Information from one's personal motor development—what went smoothly and what met obstacles and perhaps failures—is "stamped in some parts of the body."[ii]

The Feldenkrais Method is designed to retrieve and reframe such information. The method counters the forgetting of oneself, seeking to restore the functionality of movements and skeletal dynamics by eliciting sensorimotor information from the embodied memory.

Before examining how the Feldenkrais Method gains access to those memories and recollections, we shall look at two cases of scientific evidence of the memory of the organism, the sensorial, embodied memory.

---

[i] Damasio 2010, p. 144. Antonio Damasio is the David Dornsife Chair in Neuroscience, and Professor of Psychology, Philosophy, and Neurology, at the University of Southern California.

[ii] *The Potent Self*, p. xxxv.

What science says about the embodied memory

Chronic pain

An example of the body's memory and its recall that probably each of us has experienced is pain, such as headaches, which usually repeat the same sequence each time they appear. Chronic pain is more resilient and can be more severe than moderate or even intense acute pain. Chronic pain is a typical example of the body's memory. While the initial cause of pain may have been an illness, an injury, or surgery, the pain persists for a long period, even when the injury or illness has healed. Chronic pain is also a common theme among people who turn to the Feldenkrais Method for assistance.

Despite the pervasiveness of chronic pain, researchers have not come to definitive conclusions about how or why it occurs. Temporary relief is given to patients with painkillers, such as opioids and non-steroidal anti-inflammatory drugs. Research continues intensively, and notable results have been achieved by scientists around the world.[i] One worth mentioning is that of a team from King's College London. Their work provides the groundwork for an explanation of chronic pain. On the website of her laboratory, the head of the team, Dr. Franziska Denk, writes:

> Imagine if your cells kept a record of the many innumerable events that you encounter throughout your life. Each bruise or bump would leave behind a tiny molecular footprint that could then influence a cell's response at a later date.

---

[i] See Melzack and Wall, 2003

We know that this can happen: immune cells acquire "memories" and recall them when needed. This laboratory is interested in finding out whether adult nervous system cells, such as microglia and neurons, might also be able to keep similar records, specifically in the context of chronic pain.[i]

The researchers found what they were looking for. They discovered that nerve damage which occurs in the event of an accidental injury or disease can change how genes are expressed and where. Their conclusion was: "While these genes can behave normally, they do carry a memory of the initial injury."[ii]

Phantom limb

Perhaps the best example of the body's memory and its recollection is another thoroughly researched theme: the phantom limb. The case described below is evidence that the human organism harbors nonconscious reminiscences and memories, both of personal body-history and of the original template of the human body.

A phantom limb is the sensation that an amputated or missing limb is still attached. Phantom sensations may also occur after the removal of body parts other than limbs, such as a breast after mastectomy. Nearly 75 percent of individuals who have undergone an amputation experience phantom sensation in their amputated part, and the majority of the sensations are painful. People will sometimes also feel as if they are gesturing, feel itches, twitch, or even try to pick things up with an amputated hand.

---

[i] https://franziskadenk.com/research, accessed on August 24, 2021

[ii] See Denk and McMahon, 2012.

A most amazing and interesting case was reported by the neuro-scientists Vilayanur Subramanian Ramachandran and Paul McGeoch. Ramachandran has designed a simple method and device to alleviate phantom limb pain, a "mirror box." It is a box with one mirror down the center, and is used as follows. The affected limb is placed behind the mirror and kept covered, out of sight; the unaffected limb is placed symmetrically to it on the mirror side. The patient then looks into the mirror at the reflection of the intact limb and makes "mirror symmet-ric" movements, as we do when we hold palm to palm in a praying-hands gesture, or when we clap our hands. Because the subject is see-ing the reflected image of the good hand moving, it appears as if the phantom limb is also moving. Through the use of this artificial visual feedback, it becomes possible for the patient to "move" the phantom limb, and to unclench it from potentially painful positions.[i]

The noteworthy case reported by the scientists is of R. N., a 57-year-old woman who had been born with a deformed right hand, con-sisting of only three fingers and a rudimentary thumb. After a car crash at the age of 18, the woman's deformed hand was amputated, which gave rise to feelings of a phantom hand. The phantom hand was expe-rienced, however, as having all five fingers (although some of the dig-its were foreshortened). Thirty-five years after her accident, the woman was referred for treatment after her phantom hand had be-come unbearably painful. After the treatment with the "mirror box," she was able to move her phantom fingers and was relieved of pain.

---

[i] The wider use of mirrors in this way is known as mirror therapy or mirror visual feedback (MVF), and is also used in relation to brain plasticity.

Crucially, she also experienced that all five of her phantom fingers were now of normal length.[i]

Ramachandran and McGeoch stated that this case provides evidence that the brain has an innate template of a fully formed hand. In the abstract of the article published on the case, they stated that "a hardwired representation of a complete hand had always been present in her brain," but it was inhibited by a birth defect. The researchers' closing sentence is: "The case powerfully demonstrates the interaction of nature and nurture in creating and sustaining body image."[ii]

The research, thus, reveals that notwithstanding congenital anomalies, and life contingencies, the human body carries a blueprint of sorts for how the skeletal system is functionally organized at, or closest to, the optimum. It is an end product of the long evolutionary process that created and refined the human body.[iii]

How this memory can be accessed will be discussed below. First, I will show how the idea that every human being carries a memory of the template of the human body, of an optimally structured skeletal schema, can throw light on the guidelines for giving Functional Integration lessons.

---

[i] McGeoch and Ramachandran, 2012.

[ii] Ibid., p. 97.

[iii] On recent theories of memory, suggesting that the body is the medium that stimulates the sensorimotor component of remembered events, see Ianì, 2019.

Functional Integration and the body-image
Where do you start an FI? How do you do it?

Functional Integration is a hand-on modality, but the practitioner's hands act as a two-way conduit for whole-body information, enabling the teacher to perform smooth, non-invasive, and non-painful movements with the bones and articulations of the student or patient's body. This delicate and precise manual contact mirrors the student's body organization, and gently suggests different configurations that are more comfortable. During this process, the apprentice refines somatic perception, learns to reorganize the skeletal schema more clearly and efficiently, and then can discover and incorporate new movement patterns that are more pleasant and efficient.

Questions that usually arise in this context are: How do you decide where to start a lesson of FI? Which part of the body will be the first to touch and manipulate? Which one(s) will follow? How do you teach a student or patient to sharpen inner perception and to reorganize their actions more effectively? How should the practitioner assist and guide the person to reintegrate their self-image, and to initiate a process of self-change through Functional Integration lessons?

The most common answer that practitioners give is that we do not know in advance where we are going to start, or why one place is better than any other. The procedure is, first, to ask the person to make some movements, such as walking, raising a hand, or turning the head; to detect where the movement originates, what parts of the body move and which do not, the differences between the left and right sides of the body, the line of the spine, the position of the head, and so on. The idea is to get a general impression of the integration and organization of the different parts of the body in movement. We also ask about the person's practices and doings, such as the kind of work they do and the physical activities that they practice; and about any body aches and pains and their general feeling. It is only after listening and observing what the person transmits to us, both verbally and nonverbally, that the decision where to start the FI lesson is made.

Feldenkrais himself did not give much direct information about where or how to start a Functional Integration lesson. However, he did give some important clues on how to approach it. One of the clues we find in the Amherst training, where he spoke about the theme in three of the segments.[i] On these occasions, Feldenkrais touches on some of the major points of how to approach an FI lesson. He does this after giving an FI lesson to Ronnie, a woman who came in walking on crutches and in great pain, and after the lesson, left walking without crutches and with no pain.

A first point that Feldenkrais makes is that the entire approach to Functional Integration "is real improvisation"—thereby confirming that we do not know in advance where to start. Improvisation here means that the FI is done without any specific, previously prepared program. The only plan that he had in advance in Ronnie's case was not to alleviate her pain, but rather to find out what her skeletal system does that distorts her movements.

Feldenkrais explains that Functional Integration is not a question of knowing, but rather of doing: a doing guided by feeling and sensing with the hands and through the hands, to attain an attunement between the practitioner and the student. A condition is that the student must trust the practitioner, while the practitioner "must

---

[i] AM 2 – Week 3 – June 22 PM1: "Talk: FI and Knowing What to Do."
  AM 2 – Week 3 – June 23 PM1: "Talk: FI as Improvisation."
  AM 2 – Week 4 – June 29 PM1: "Talk: About FI."

be a very mature person," with a high level of somatic awareness. Attunement is understood as kinesthetic and sensorial experiencing of the other, a feeling of reciprocal connectedness. In essence, the idea is to engage in a conversation without spoken language between the practitioner and the student or patient, but rather a communication by touch and movement, a haptic communication.

Another clue we get from a recording of the neuroscientist Karl Pribram reporting on an encounter that he had with Feldenkrais and the anthropologist Margaret Mead. On that occasion Mead asked Feldenkrais about his method in general and Functional Integration in particular, "How do you do it?" This was Feldenkrais's answer, as told by Pribram:

> When I see a person I know how they should be, they should look, I see the perfect person when I see I know how you are and how you ought to be, they are all in one, but how you ought to be is right there, and then I simply go to work, I have my techniques, and try this and try that, it is not very well structured, it doesn't really matter whether I start with a little toe, an ear, the neck, or whatever until I get that person to look like the person that I think they ought to be, and I know exactly how they ought to look.[i]

The "how you are" and "how you ought to be" is the blending of the two images that Feldenkrais perceives: the image of the person lying on the table, and the image of how that specific body could be lying on the table if it was fully functionally organized. Feldenkrais perceives

---

[i] Pribram's keynote address to the 1987 North American Guild Conference is included in "The Feldenkrais–Pribram Discussions."

the uniqueness of the body and at the same time the template of the human body schema composed by the five cardinal lines, including the smallest details of the skeletal system and the flow of movement through it. It is through this perspective that the approach to giving Ronnie, or anyone else, a Functional Integration lesson becomes clearer. The idea is to find out what the skeletal system does that distorts the movements by blending the two body schemas.

Here we find encapsulated once again a main aim of the Feldenkrais Method, which is to preserve the uniqueness and singularity of each body assemblage while at the same time bringing into being a functionally integrated body based on the skeletal system shared by all members of the human species. In the adequate blending of these two, every individual can acquire a functional body and its equivalent self-image.

PART TWO

SELF-CHANGE

THEORY AND PRACTICE

4

The Principles for Self-Transformation

Self-transformation rests on revisiting and resetting the different chapters of the history of the personal body, which means to bring to the surface somatic memories both of sensorimotor development, and of the pathways of movements that shape skeletal dynamics across a lifetime. The question that arises is whether and how it is possible to do that. Feldenkrais is confident, and in full agreement with Damasio that "All of our memories ... exist in our brains in dispositional form, waiting to become explicit images or actions."[i] Feldenkrais asserts that "many of the most useful things that we have learned in early childhood from the moment of conception and through our life... are dormant in our brain somewhere until they are necessary. Then you can evoke them."[ii]

There are different ways to access information about experiences human beings have gone through during their infancy or after. One of

---

[i] Damasio 2010, p. 144.

[ii] *Feldenkrais: Professional Training Program Transcript.* Amherst. Week One. p.6.

them, and the most common, is the psychological one in any of its variants. Feldenkrais valued Freud's work and psychoanalysis; however, he was aware of its shortcomings as well.[i] On several occasions, he expressed the limits of language, a central feature and tool of psychoanalysis and of all types of verbal psychotherapy, as a means to access and retrieve information from the nonconscious or subconscious.

> One of the great disadvantages of the spoken language is the fact that it permits us to become estranged from our real selves to such an extent that we often have the mistaken belief that we have imagined something, or thought of something, where in reality we have only recalled the appropriate word.[ii]

Having access to words that describe feelings related to sensorimotor development does not necessarily make the full experiences available. Language might misrepresent personal feelings, since it "forces everybody to sense in the same way… when, in fact, we are all different."[iii] An underlying idea of the Feldenkrais Method is that, given that primal sensations and feelings originated in the preverbal time, they can be accessed, perhaps exclusively, through nonverbal methods. Specifically, accessing sensorimotor information acquired in the past—from the moment of conception through motor development, and at other junctures of personal life—should be done through a sensorimotor practice. In Feldenkrais's words, "I believe… that sensory

---

[i] For a more detailed account of Feldenkrais's opinion and attitude on Freud and psychoanalysis, see Reese 2015, chaps. 6–7.

[ii] *Awareness Through Movement*, p.135.

[iii] 1974 *London ATM Workshop*, p. 9.

stimuli are closer to our unconscious, subconscious, or autonomous functioning than any of our conscious understanding." [i]

I found that the Feldenkrais Method accesses the sensorimotor nonconscious through the assemblage of the following three principles, and their corresponding strategies.

Revisiting the organization and patterns of the primary movements

This is done by reproducing all the different steps involved in the process of learning how to roll, sit up, crawl, stand up, and walk, thereby recapitulating, assimilating, and adjusting anew the original patterns of sensorimotor development (chapter 5).

Replication of prenatal and early life reflexes

Primitive reflexes are the building blocks of motor development, and their integration is essential for sensorimotor and cognitive growth. By replicating them, along with the different steps of motor development that they give rise to, the Feldenkrais Method revitalizes their integration (chapter 6).

---

[i] *The Elusive Obvious*, p. 3. The term "subconscious" is used in psychology to refer to the part of the mind that we are not fully aware of. The term "unconscious" is a term coined by Freud to refer to parts of the mind that cannot be known by the conscious mind, and that include desires, traumatic memories, and painful emotions that have been repressed. During the last decades, neuroscience uses "nonconscious," and "nonconsciousness," to refer to the processes relevant to maintaining life without being consciously recognized. Feldenkrais uses "subconscious" and "unconscious" and not the later "nonconscious," but his use of "autonomous functioning" encompasses the nonconscious processes that neuroscientists refer to.

Resetting and renewal of habitual movements

Habitual movements regulate significant functions and capacities of body movements and of character and behavior. While contributing to a smoother running of life, habitual movements can become automatized or even compulsive, causing tension and pain, and affecting the way we feel with ourselves. The method demonstrates alternative ways to do the same action, thereby disassembling rooted habitual patterns and reattuning ourselves to the process of self-change (chapter 7).

We shall notice that practicing the Feldenkrais Method is largely an enjoyable experience. While some lessons can be demanding in flexibility and athleticism, most do not require great physical effort and are built on the idea that the movements should be easy, painless, intriguing, slow, and pleasurable, thereby facilitating awareness and neutralizing the achievement mindset prevalent in most body practices. But then again, reproducing patterns of motor development and learning may give rise to obstacles. These can be motor-related or associated with other layers of embodied experience, such as affects and feelings, causing frustration and disappointment.

The Feldenkrais Method teaches how to overcome those obstacles by offering alternative ways of doing the movement. Walking, sitting in a chair, lifting an object, raising a hand, rolling the head, can be done in different ways by the same individual. Some ways might be more comfortable than others, some will need more effort than others, but having alternative ways to do the same action enhances the integration of the skeletal system. Moreover, by having alternative ways to do every day habitual actions, the participant becomes aware of their capacity to change, thereby giving a nuanced, better-attuned perspective to the self-image.

5

Reproducing the Motor Development Chain

The way motor development takes shape in every individual—from rolling to sitting up, to crawling, to standing up, and to walking—resonates later in life in their movements and posture. Indeed, the onset of balancing and rolling is a developmental transition that sets in motion a cascade of changes across a range of domains: motor, sensory, emotional, and cognitive, including social interactions and language learning. The Feldenkrais Method reenacts the chain of movements of motor development to bring to the surface sensorimotor moments and processes archived in the organism, and encoded in the nervous system and brain, to restore functionality.

Motor development is a process that evolves from primitive and early-life reflexes that are active during the fetal stage and the first months of life after birth. Accomplishment in each stage of the process depends on the successful completion of the previous one. This means that every time an infant masters a new skill or ability, that mastery directly enables the next level of skill development. Balancing enables rolling.

Rolling enables sitting up. Sitting enables crawling. Crawling enables standing up, which enables "cruising"—stepping sideways while holding on to furniture. Cruising enables walking, which enables running.

In many cases, and for different reasons, infants might not fully master one of the movements of the process and still go to the next step. An infant could do the movement of rolling while leaving a small gap in the full mastery of the movement and still manage to sit up, crawl, stand up on two feet, and walk. Infants could even skip steps without it preventing them from accomplishing the next step. There are, for instance, infants who do not crawl, but go from sitting to standing. While this is considered to be a normal variation, missing a step might resonate in the mobility of the person at a later age. In severe cases, and when there is also a delay in other phases of development, it can cause some difficulties in motor and sensory faculties. In mild cases, it could affect posture and, for example, make it difficult to play some sport. The aim of the Feldenkrais Method is not to transform every one of us into accomplished athletes, but rather to restore functionality and to integrate the skeletal system and body movements.

Functionality is restored by reproducing the chain of motor development unabridged. The idea is to replicate the movements of each stage of the process to fill in the gaps, if there were any—and there usually are, in all of us—that might have been left in the original process that the person went through. Practicing the method sparks awareness of the sequence of the process of constructing the movements and postures, reintegrating them into the body schema.

In the following section, I present a selection of exemplary lessons that reproduce the path of motor development and retrace the initial moments when the movements were performed and configured.

The Lessons

Balancing and rolling

Rolling is a crucial milestone of motor and sensorial development. Rolling is the first experience of moving the entire body, and it starts the process of coping with balance by using the weight of different parts of the body as a lever to roll. By stimulating coordination, rolling helps to shape the balance mechanism for varying orientations in the field of gravity, which is a building block for crawling, sitting up, standing up, and walking.

At the sensorial level, rolling fosters the internal sense of the body and how to move its different parts to achieve a goal. Rolling stimulates proprioception, assisting the body in sensing where the body parts are relative to the ground, to each other, and to the space and objects around it. This internal sense helps to navigate the near environment and adapt to information received through the external senses, as the infant experiences objects and surfaces of different textures, temperatures, and densities.

The following set of lessons that have the movement of rolling as their main motif aims at a sensorial recollection of those primary motor experiences. The lessons explore how balance responds to the force of gravity, and facilitate the adjustment and reorganization of *acture* by showing how movement is generated using the weight of some parts of the body, rather than the strength of the muscles.[i]

AY 313: Rolling at the Rate of Stretching and Bending – (Reel 21/4/1)

This lesson is a perfect place to begin the reenactment of the most basic, primary movements. The lesson reproduces the fetal position and a primitive reflex to experiment with balance and to demonstrate how to roll effortlessly from the back to the stomach and back.

From the fetal position, lying on one side and on the back, the knees and elbows are flexed and brought toward each other, then moved apart by lengthening the limbs and the back, allowing the head to arch backward. The slow and continuous movement generates an unfolding, outward-growing force that moves the body through a curved path and gradually rolls it until a full roll onto the back or stomach is completed. The extension and flexion of the arms, and the movement of the back and the head, reproduce the Moro reflex (chapter 6).

AY 122: Rolling Right and Left – (Reel 9/3/1)

As in the preceding lesson, it is the dynamism generated by rocking the body and lengthening the arms and

---

[i] The word "acture" is used by Feldenkrais as a synthesis of action and posture, as a dynamic posture.

legs, rather than the strength of the muscles, that facilitates rolling effortlessly.

Lying face up, the movement is initiated and aided by the push of a standing foot that rolls the body to the side, and the lengthening of the opposite arm along the floor overhead. The hip is lifted by the pushing foot, and the shoulder on the same side is added as an active point in the rolling. Lying face down, raising the hip on one side and bending and drawing up that knee rolls the body smoothly to the back. The arm moving away from the center of the body is a feature of the Asymmetrical Tonic Neck Reflex, ATNR (chapter 6).[i]

Practicing these lessons and experiencing how the lengthening and the weight of the limbs produce rolling movements, the participants become sensorially aware of the dynamism of their skeletal system.

Some people could see these two lessons as supporting the idea that there is an advantage in mostly laying infants on their backs, rather than on their bellies. The reason is that lying face up it is possible to roll without the need to use the strength of the muscles, which in infants are not yet strong enough to do the movement by themselves.

AY 542.2: *Baby Rolls – (Reel 35/4/2)* [ii]

This lesson reenacts the moments in early life when, by moving the whole body gently to and fro, the infant first

---

[i] A video of this lesson by Ute Müller is at https://feldynotebook. com/rolling-right-and-left-ay-122/?cn-reloaded=1.

[ii] This lesson is not included in the Alexander Yanai Collections.

learns how to roll and turn from the back to the stomach and back. The objective is to replicate initial moments of motor development that most people go through in their infancy.

The lesson stages the body rocking up and down in two baby positions. Lying face down, the hands close to the head, the gaze and the head are raised and lowered, helped by bending the knees. Lying face up, with the legs and the arms half bent and the fists close to the mouth "like a baby," the head is raised while the elbows and knees flex and extend, coming close to and apart from each other. With a slight rocking to the sides, and using the weight of one hip and the straightening of one leg, the body rolls until it lies on the stomach and then rolls back again. The contact of the back and the chest with the floor prompts awareness of how gravitation is experienced, and how it affects movement.

AY 178: Lengthening the Arms – (Reel 13/1/2)

This lesson outlines the axis of rotation by marking the diagonal lines of the body. Lying on the back with one arm extended above the head, pressing the floor with the sole of the opposite standing foot elongates the arm and generates a slight rolling of the body to the side. While rolling, the attention follows the movement that travels diagonally, from the foot to the hip joint, to the lumbar spine, across the midline to the opposite clavicle, shoulder, arm, and hand. The lengthening movements are repeated lying face down and sitting.

Rolling to sit

The process of rolling to sitting up usually has its earliest rudiments in the first month of life, and comes to fruition around the sixth month. The following lessons reproduce the movements from rolling to sitting up, by disassembling the act of sitting up to its components and showing how an organized skeletal system can sit effortlessly.

AY 327: Sitting – Lying, Continuation – (Reel 22/3/3)

This lesson organizes the body to sit from rolling, without actually sitting up. The lesson breaks down to its basic components the movement of half rolling to the side, bringing the body to a near sitting position. The objective is to smoothly roll to the side, moved by the weight of the different parts of the body, rather than by contracting the stomach and neck muscles.

Lying face up, with the legs bent and feet not touching the floor, the head raised, and the hands interlaced holding the back of the head, or lifted in a loose circle in front, rocking back and forth and left and right, and rolling the hip and the shoulders to the sides while stretching out a leg, the body comes close to a sitting position. The way to do it is by softening the thorax and the lateral ribs so that they do not obstruct the body from rolling.

The idea of this lesson is to dynamize the body to a side-forward-bending, near-sitting position, helped by the lifting-rolling movement that is amplified by the weight of the head, shoulders, hip, and leg, and the softening of the chest, rather than by muscular effort.

AY 003: Rolling to Sit with the Elbows – (Reel 1/2/2)
AY 223: Rolling from the Back to Side-Sitting –
(Reel 16/1/2)

These two almost identical lessons, like the previous one, dissect to its minute pieces how, from the supine position, rolling over to the side brings the body to sit up.[i]

The sequence of movements in AY 003 is a continuation of the lesson above (AY 327), though here the elbows and the hands are more active. A hand holds and lifts the head, directs it to the right and then to the left side continuously, bringing the elbow close to the floor until it touches it. The other arm, extended downward on the floor at about a 45-degree angle to the side, supports the body on its elbow when the body rises to the side, easing the side rolling and bringing the body to half-sitting, and finally to sitting up. The use of the elbow retraces a stage in motor development when infants use their elbows to come to sit and to break falls.

The side sitting in AY 223 is done by holding the head and lifting it with the hands, and then with one hand, rolling to the side while bending. The movement is facilitated by lowering the elbow of the arm holding the head toward the floor while rolling onto the other elbow. Then, releasing the head, raising that arm toward

---

[i] A couple of short videos of "Rolling to Sit with the Elbows" can be accessed in Feldy Notebook: https://feldynotebook.com/rolling-to-sit-with-the-elbows-ay3/. For the importance of side sitting in this context, see Shelhav 2019, chapter 6.

the ceiling, and using it as a lever to help the body turn, while bending both knees at once, generates a rotational momentum that brings the body to side sitting, from one side to the other. (The reversal of this lesson is AY 417, chapter 8.)

One of the movements that facilitate rolling for newborns is the flexing and extending of the arms and legs, as in the lesson AY 178 above. Certainly, flexing and extending the arms and the legs are crucial to the survival mechanism of *Homo sapiens*—they are movements that could be used to reach fruit hanging from a tree, to reach and grasp a branch of the tree to stay safe from a predator, to hold the breast of the mother to be fed, and to reach an object lying close enough to be picked up. To be sure, flexing and extending arms and legs are auxiliary movements present in all the steps of motor development, from rolling to walking.

AY 067: Lengthening the Leg Into Pulling Movements While Rolling – (Reel 5/4/1)

This lesson, Feldenkrais says, is a "perfect rolling of the body that brings it to sitting up without effort and strength." Indeed, the lesson stages in a very clear fashion how sitting up can grow naturally from a regular and steady rolling, by incorporating the extremities into the movement.

Lying face up and holding one foot by the outer edge of the sole with that hand from between the legs, it is by flexing and extending while raising and swinging the arm and leg in the direction of the same-side shoulder that the rolling movement is initiated. Essentially, the coordinated movements of the leg and the arm bring the body from rolling to sitting up effortlessly. It becomes easy to swing and roll from one side to the other. (The reversal of this lesson is E 35/Es 33, chapter 8.)

AM 1 – Week 2 – June 16 AM2: Rolling With Entire Self
The most important theme that Feldenkrais refers to in this lesson, and relevant for all the lessons in this section, is simultaneity. Doing the movements simultaneously makes the effortless rolling still easier.

The rolling movement starts when lying on one side, and taking the bent leg and arm of the other side away from and toward one another simultaneously. The quality of simultaneity is improved by shifting the attention to the connection between the hand and the foot, the knee and the elbow, and the hip and shoulder, all moving closer to and apart from each other. For the participant, the lesson improves coordination of the movements, which echoes a higher integration of the skeletal system.

Crawling

Crawling is a vital movement in the motor development of human beings. Crawling involves motor, sensory, emotional, and cognitive aspects. In the Feldenkrais Method we find lessons that stage the beginnings of crawling in every person, as well as the archaic origins of crawling in human beings.

The archaic roots, Feldenkrais reminds us, we find in the movements of fish in water, in those of the first amphibians that left the water to live on land, and in the crawling of reptiles, such as lizards and alligators. Feldenkrais refers to the prehistoric roots of crawling in "Fish Swimming" (AY 512), "Reptiles" (AY 513), and "Walking and Crawling" (AY 502). The blueprint of the origins of crawling, from which walking in human beings evolved, is well ingrained in the human brain and nervous system. It is part of the evolutionary history and body-sensorial memory of humankind. The lessons staging those movements aim to reproduce and take hold of evolutionary moments in motor development to enliven the most basic and rudimentary patterns of crawling.

For each human being, crawling is a major step in their motor and sensory development. It is the position in which an infant will be putting weight on his/her hands through the long bones of the arms for the first time, developing strength and stability at the shoulders. Crawling improves coordination by facilitating the working together of the left and right sides of the body, thereby bridging the right and left hemispheres of the brain. At the sensorial level, crawling sparks body awareness of space, helping to fine-tune the vestibular balance apparatus. Consequently, crawling helps to enhance depth perception and the sense of touch. At the emotional and cognitive levels, crawling is the first movement that enables the infant to independently move and reach for objects, playing with toys and bringing them to the mouth. The Symmetrical Tonic Neck Reflex (STNR, chapter 6), also known as the crawling reflex, is a steppingstone on which crawling is assembled.

There are several ways in which infants may crawl, though three of them are considered to be the main ones: belly crawling, scooting, and crisscross crawling. The three always come in the same order, though some infants may skip one of them.[i]

Belly crawling

Belly crawling, also known as the commando crawl, is the way the majority of infants begin crawling and start to move independently. The infants keep their abdomen, their tummy, against the floor as they move along by pushing with the legs. In this style of crawling, infants do not yet get up on their hands and knees, which requires greater strength and balance.

AY 099: Lifting the Elbows With a Loose Hand –
(Reel 8/1/3)

This lesson stages the first movements of the developmental process that facilitates infants to start creeping and crawling. The lesson's objective is to organize and ease the lifting of the head, which is the first and necessary movement to start crawling.

Lying with the face down, with a leg bent at the knee on the floor at 90 degrees, the arms on the floor, bent above the head, by raising the elbows—one, then the other, then together—the shoulder girdle and the cervical spine soften and are integrated with the movement of the head. For the participant, this lesson can be highly beneficial by adjusting the organization of the upper spine and carriage of the head.

---

[i] See AM 1 – Week 2 – June 20 AM1: "Talk: Crawling and Brain Functions."

AY 515: Dragging Knees to the Stomach – (Reel 33/4/1)
This lesson stages the movements of the legs that are necessary for belly crawling. Lying face up and face down, the lesson effects coordination of the movement of the knees bending alternately to the sides, dragging each one toward the stomach on the floor, with other movements of the body, such as the hip lifting and pelvis turning to the side, and extending and dragging the arm in an arc overhead so it comes under the head to the other side. The movements of the legs combined with those of the hips slightly turn the body to the sides, in an oscillatory movement that is part of crawling on the stomach.

AY 512: Fish Swimming – (Reel 33/3/3)
This lesson is similar to and a continuation of the one above, and seeks to improve the coordination of the movements of the legs with the hands and head for belly crawling.

Lying face down, belly crawling is built bit by bit, paying attention to all the details necessary to crawl. Included are the bending of each knee sideways, the movement of the head from side to side, dragging an arm, and bringing it to a standing position close to the head. In the end, all the parts come together, making belly crawling one simple movement.

Scooting

Scooting is another first style of crawling for infants, and it is done by sitting up and scooting along on their bottoms. The infants use their legs to power themselves across the floor. A variant of this form of crawling is when the infant powers him/herself on one leg while dragging the other leg. In this mode, the infant's bottom bears the weight, while the torso is in an upright position.

AY 513: Reptiles – (Reel 33/3/4)

This lesson compiles the movements developed in the above three lessons to facilitate standing up and walking, with the purpose of understanding "how walking was initially shaped."

The lesson perfects the harmonization of the movements of arms, legs, hips, and head necessary for crawling in the different styles, which are staged with movements corresponding to each one of them. For belly-crawling it coordinates between the movement of the arms with the feet dragging on the floor, and pushing with the toes and ball of the foot to advance. For crawling that is similar to the swimming of a fish, both hands move in unison forward and backward. When crawling "like a lizard," the coordination is between the arm and leg of each side, which move together. There is also crawling as scooting, by sitting and dragging the body forward with the hands, while the feet and knees are on the floor. In crisscross crawling, each arm and the opposite leg move simultaneously.

Crisscross crawling

Crisscross crawling is done by moving forward an arm and the opposite leg in unison. This is the last step before infants stand up and begin walking. This style of crawling helps the infant to cross the midline of the body that divides it between right and left. It is thus important for brain development, since it bridges the right and left hemispheres of the brain, allowing electrical impulses (information) to pass freely between the two. This development is key for physical coordination and to increase bone and muscle strength. A building block of this movement is the STNR crawling reflex (chapter 6). The following lessons are a preamble for well-organized crisscross crawling.

AY 057: Lifting the Head on All Fours – (Reel 4/4/2)

Lifting the head is an essential movement for motor development and body control. The ability to hold the head still, lift it to either side, and turn it is the basis for rolling over, sitting up, and reaching an upright posture. In this lesson the movement is incorporated into crawling.

The lesson organizes the body to crawl on all fours. While standing on the hands and knees, the ability to arch the spine and raise the head improves without much muscular effort from the neck, but rather with the movement of the waist. The movements of the lumbar spine are integrated into those of the head and gaze, which is indispensable for crawling on all fours. The difference between the upper and lower part of the body is underscored, while the movements of flexion and extension of the neck activate far- and near-distance vision. This lesson reenacts movements from the STNR and the Moro Reflex.

AY 123: On the Knees; Diagonal See-Saw – (Reel 9/3/6)

This lesson marks the two diagonal lines that are at play in crisscross crawling. It plugs into the sensorimotor connection between an arm and the leg of the opposite side, which is needed for crawling on all fours.

Lying face down, the seesaw movement is generated by raising and lowering the head and arm of one side and the leg from the opposite side. The swinging movements are done both lying face down and standing on knees and elbows/forearms.

E 27: Primitive Locomotion: Coordinating the Locomotive Joints/Es 25: Crawling, on Knees

The movements of this lesson assist in organizing crisscross crawling, even though there is no crisscross crawling as we know it.

Standing on hands and knees, the sequence includes moving the hip back towards sitting on the heels, sliding a foot between the opposite hand and knee to side sit, and moving the head and the gaze up and down. The movements are done in different variations: first one foot does the movement, then the other, then they alternate. The head is raised and lowered with every movement, elongating and shortening the spine. Crawling is done in a non-habitual way, crossing one leg through in front of the other leg, underscoring the diagonal lines of the movement.

The lesson softens the hip joints, the spine, and gives more mobility to the pelvis. Feldenkrais says that "When you do this movement, the spine, from the pelvis to the neck, is twisting in every movement, bending also, and making the spine more flexible." These qualities are indispensable for crisscross crawling, and to increase the range of mobility in general.

AY 528: Advancing on All Fours – (Reel 34/3/2)
This lesson seeks to improve the ability to kneel hands-free from the floor, which is the preliminary movement for standing up. Like in the lesson above, it makes use of non-habitual movements, such as threading one leg through the space between the opposite hand and knee and kneeling with the legs crossed. The purpose of the non-familiar movements is to activate and integrate other parts of the body into kneeling instead of putting the hand on the floor for support.

Standing to walk

There is no consensus among the scientific community as to why the genus *Homo* started walking upright. Some of the explanations put forward for bipedalism are: (a) Humans could free hands for increased tool use or for weapons in hunting, or the for the use of containers to transport plant foods obtained by gathering. (b) Bipedalism evolved from the need to avoid predators, as a higher head facilitates seeing longer distances over the grassland. (c) Natural selection favored bipedalism in open environments because it decreases exposure to the sun and helps keep the brain cool. (d) Recent research suggests that bipedalism in humans may have come from foraging in treetops.

It is reasonable to think that a combination of some of these factors might be at the base of that development. Whatever the cause(s) may be, bipedalism represents a fundamental step in the evolution of the human species, and the faculty exists in every person. What was developed and learned over a long period of time by the human species can be achieved in less than a year by most individuals.

The following lessons, which have walking as their main theme, are actual preparations for walking by improving posture and adjusting the distribution of the weight of the body on the heels, which are necessary features for walking.[i]

The posture rarely changes, says Feldenkrais in AY 234: you can recognize someone from a far distance by their posture and by the way they stand and walk. The objective of the following series of three lessons is, indeed, to experiment with changes in weight distribution, support of the body, and the pull of gravity, fashioning a better acture and comfortable walking.

> *AY 234: Standing Backward, #1 – (Reel 17/1/1)*
> *AY 238: Standing Backward, #2 – (Reel 17/2/1)*
> *AY 235: Standing (Shaking in the Heels – (Reel 17/1/2)*
> In these lessons, acture is improved by moving different
> parts of the body backward while standing, exploring
> the point of gravity of the body and its support on the
> feet. In AY 234 and AY 238 it is the pelvis that moves

---

[i] On bipedalism and gravity, see Le Huec et al. 2011.

backward, first in the center, then to one side, and then to the other side. Putting the weight on the heels, the shoulder girdle joins the backward movements, then the waist, and then the back of the head. These movements change the fulcrum—the pivot point of support in the foot. The lessons also experiment with changing the support of the body from one heel to the other. The attention is on the way the weight shifts to one leg and its heel.

Lesson AY 235 repeats the basic movements of the other two and develops them further, adding backward movements of other parts of the body, such as the knees, the middle of the back at the height of the shoulders, the ribs, and the neck. It also shakes the heels, bouncing them on the floor, stimulating them, and through them, stimulates the long bones that carry our weight. AY 235 and AY 238 experiment with shifting weight from heel to heel with the feet standing both parallel and crossed, and with the pelvis moving in an arc.

AY 274: Introduction to Walking 1 – (Reel 19/2/4)
AY 275: Introduction to Walking 2, Continuation – (Reel 19/2/5)

These lessons prepare for walking, with a focus on the sense of balance, weight distribution on the left and right foot and heels, and breathing.

The sense of balance is explored by shifting the weight from one foot to the other—essential to walking—moving the pelvis in an arc. The weight shifts from heel to heel in various configurations of the feet, such as crossed, uncrossed, and lifting the forefoot. In AY 275 the neck region and the trunk move independently of the head and pelvis, coupled with an examination of the impact that these movements have on balance.

AY 502: *Walking and Crawling – (Reel 33/1/2)*

This lesson stimulates awareness in walking movements and reorganizes acture by combining habitual with non-habitual walking and crawling.

In habitual walking, arms and legs from opposite sides move in unison. In this lesson the habitual movements alternate with the non-habitual movements: having the arm and leg of the same side moving forward and backward in concert. The habitual/non-habitual sequence is also performed crawling on all fours, crawling on the stomach pushing with elbows and knees, and crawling on the back. Attention in non-habitual walking is on the amplified rotational movement of the hips, the head, and the shoulders. Other non-habitual movements in walking experimented with in this lesson are bringing the back of the body backward, in a "monkey walk" with the back and the knees bent; and walking moving the chin forward, like a bird pecking. The non-habitual movements seek to incorporate those parts of the body that are inactive or not sensed in each specific case (chapter 7).

AY 501: Introduction to Walking – (Reel 33/1/1)

As in the lesson above, non-habitual elements of walking alternate with habitual walking to improve acture. The lesson starts with slow walking in a non-habitual way, moving an arm and a leg of the same side in unison, while attending to the movement of the hips and shoulders and the effects they have on the feet while walking. The lesson introduces other non-habitual elements that alternate with habitual walking, such as taking one hip back, then taking it forward while walking without moving the arms; and bending the head sideways, bringing the ear close to the shoulder. These movements aim to explore the effects of the force of gravity on posture while in movement.

The chain of sensorimotor development that begins with rolling as a first movement of the newborn and culminates after approximately one year in walking is a product of transforming non-voluntary movements into voluntary ones, thereby shaping the functionality of the body's motion. Voluntary movements have their origin in non-voluntary reflexes, some of them already active in the womb, others becoming active in the early months of life. In the following chapter, we will examine how the Feldenkrais Method incorporates these involuntary movements into the process of self-transformation.

6

Reflexes as Archives

A reflex is a rapid movement evoked in response to a stimulus. Often, reflexes do not involve the brain and are involuntary and unconscious actions, like the *reflex arc*: a special type of neural circuit that begins with a sensory neuron at a receptor and ends with a motor neuron at an effector. An example is pulling the hand away upon inadvertently getting very close to something hot. The automatic response is caused by an electrical impulse that travels up the arm to the spinal cord and is relayed back to the muscles, which contract.[i]

But reflexes are more than electrical impulses traveling through the nervous system. Reflexes are archives of information that regulate actions and reactions for life management, including survival, self-preservation, and adjustment. When needed, the information etched in the organism is evoked, accompanied by action.

---

[i] Reflexes that produce a quick, automatic response to a stimulus are also known as *phasic*. In contrast, reflexes that show slow, steady-state contractions are known as *tonic*.

Primitive and early-life reflexes are building blocks of motor development, part of the heritage that evolution has bestowed on all human beings. Rolling, sitting up, crawling, and standing up evolve from those reflexes. Primitive reflexes can be prenatal or articulated in the early weeks or months of the newborn's life; as the infant grows and develops, the reflexes are suppressed. When infantile reflexes are not properly and fully integrated and remain active, body parts cannot move independently, which can lead to delay in some aspects of development. Indeed, incomplete integration of the reflexes can be mild or severe. In extreme cases it can contribute to anxiety and learning disorders. In mild cases, it can affect posture, balance, coordination, or sensory perception.[i]

The Feldenkrais Method includes lessons designed to reframe the primitive reflexes, recreating the movements from their inception and retrieving the steps of the process whereby involuntary movements become voluntary. The aim in view, however, is not to reinstate the reflex itself—which is neither possible nor necessary—but rather to awaken sensorial elements of the movements, and elicit information from personal body-history to reintegrate their functionality. The idea is to bring to the surface nonconscious schemas of action and, eventually, to revivify cerebral maps and neuronal connections.

The Lessons

The importance that primitive reflexes have in the Feldenkrais Method can be appreciated by looking at the lesson that Feldenkrais

---

[i] See Easton, 1972, Kamm et al. 1990.

chose to open the renowned Amherst training course: "Sucking – Life's First Movement."

Sucking is a reflex that begins in utero. After birth, when the roof of the mouth is touched, the infant will begin to suck. Unlike other newborn reflexes, the sucking reflex doesn't disappear, but by four months of age it becomes a voluntary action. The sucking reflex is important for survival, since an infant who cannot suck and coordinate sucking with swallowing and breathing will have difficulty with feeding. Feldenkrais refers to the mouth as the organ through which "awareness of the outside world originates," [i] and so sucking is a movement that is crucial not only for survival but for connection and discovery.

AM 1 – Week 1 – June 9 AM1:
Sucking – Life's First Movement

In this lesson, Feldenkrais instructs the participants, "Now, go so slowly, make the movement so slow as if you do it for the first time in your life."

The idea here is that conscious sucking, the reenactment of this primary reflex, might restore a dormant or effaced connection in the brain or nervous system. The aim is to bring sensorimotor information from the unconscious to consciousness, with the intent to revive the process and the instant when the reflex became a voluntary action.

---

[i] "Image, Movement, and Actor," p. 118.

Asymmetrical tonic neck reflex (ATNR)

When infants lie on their back and turn the head to one side, the arm and leg of the side the head is facing stretch out, and the opposite arm and leg bend up. The ATNR, which is often called the "fencing" reflex, is most prominent at one month of age and disappears around the sixth month. The reflex may remain available later in life, providing a built-in pattern that can be called upon as necessary.[i]

The functional significance of the ATNR is wide-ranging. During birth, the reflex helps the infant in the womb turn and twist to navigate the birth canal. In the weeks that follow, it enables the infant to observe his/her hand, thereby facilitating the development of hand-eye coordination. This feature facilitates dividing the body in half vertically—into left and right sides—triggering the development of the nervous system and brain. The ATNR is also present about the time an infant begins rolling over from back to stomach competently and regularly. It is thought that this reflex helps prevent the infant from rolling over onto his/her stomach before the brain and body are ready.[ii] The following lessons reproduce the main components of the reflex.

AY 068: Rolling the Fists – (Reel 5/4/2)

Lying face up, with the arms extended at the height of the shoulders and the hands curled into loose fists, both fists are rolled upward (supination: thumb toward the

---

[i] See Higgins 1991, Henderson et al. 1993.

[ii] Researchers argue that when the ATNR is retained, there are developmental delays that could present themselves after infancy. Some of the issues include poor hand-eye coordination, difficulty with visual tracking and with handwriting. Dyslexia has also been linked to the retention of this reflex.

ceiling) and downward (pronation: thumb toward the floor) simultaneously; then they are rolled in opposite directions, until the "upward" arm reaches like a fencer lunging with the foil. This movement is buttressed by turning the head to the side of the "upward" hand, lifting the opposite shoulder and hip from the floor. The arms are also extended to the sides and the fists rolled in the sitting position, in synchrony with the turn of the head from side to side.

For infants, the movement of the arms toward and away from the body teaches the brain where the vertical midline is localized. The midline is important in the control of the body for coordination and balance, but more significantly represents maturation of the communication within the brain. Communication from one side of the brain to the other is necessary for processing and interpretation of the sounds babies hear and the images they see. In this lesson, the turn of the head toward the rolling-upward arm reactivates eye-hand contact.

Feldenkrais calls the movement of one fist rolling up and the other down "the fencing position." A similar lesson given in the San Francisco training carries the name of Errol Flynn, the legendary actor portraying an undefeated fencer in his most famous films.[i]

---

[i] Lesson 6: "Rolling Arms, Rolling Fists, Errol Flynn," in *San Francisco Evening Class Notes.*

A group of lessons that reproduce the main features of the ATNR focuses on the vertical midline of the body fashioned by an extended arm and extended leg, which are lengthened and move away from the center of the body.

> ***AY 322: In Sitting, Lengthening the Arms – (Reel 22/2/2)***
> In this lesson, the body is extended and lengthened by moving arms and legs toward and away from the body, underscoring the midline.
>
> In the sitting position, the legs are straight and comfortably spread; at first with the support of one hand on the floor behind, the other arm is extended, above and parallel to the leg on the same side, about 45 degrees from the center. The arm reaches and lengthens forward, and the opposite side of the pelvis lifts from the floor, amplifying the lengthening movement. The movement of the arm, now starting in the hip, connects with the pelvis and the sit bones (*ischial tuberosities*) through the spine. Gradually variations on the movement are introduced: extending the arm straight forward, and over the opposite leg; lifting one and then the other sit bone, while holding the head still; extending one arm forward and the other backward. Turning the head in each extending movement brings the hand-eye connection into play, and integrates the upper spine and shoulders into the movement. The body finally stretches and lengthens in a highly integrated movement and with maximum reach.

The diagonal lines facilitate differentiating between the left and the right side of the body, a function that enables perceptual and cognitive development by marking the division of the brain into two hemispheres. The following lessons plug into that feature.

AY 345: Diagonal Image – (Reel 23/3/4)

The ATNR divides the body in half vertically, into left and right sides, triggering the development of an infant's nervous system and brain. In this lesson, this motif is activated. The differentiation between the two sides is done by distinguishing between parts of the body—shoulder, leg, hip—on each side. The resonance of this differentiation with the five-line image is a theme of the lesson as well.

Lying face up, the string of movements includes bending a leg and bringing it close to the chest while the other heel pushes downward; lengthening an arm above the head while the other arm, close to the body, extends downward; and combining the movements of the arms and legs. These are slow and gradual movements, exploring and cultivating sensorial awareness of each side of the body, the spine, and the five-line self-image.

AY 112: A Plane Dividing the Body #1 – (Reel 9/1/3)
AY 115: A Plane Dividing the Body #2 – (Reel 9/1/6)

These lessons revivify body lateralization, which is at the basis of primitive reflexes, specifically ATNR, STNR, and TLR. Lateralization is here attained by using imagination to visualize and perceive the midline of the body that divides it into left and right, and to explore how it differs from the "real" midline.

The lateralization is generated by an imaginary ball slowly moving and drawing a plane that divides the body along the middle line. The ball rolls slowly from the bridge of the nose down and up along the whole body, from head to feet. The ball goes between the legs, the buttocks, and up the spine, until it closes a complete circle. Then the ball bounces, creating an imaginary plane that goes from the ceiling to the floor, cutting through the body at the midline.

Another group of lessons that reproduce the main features of the ATNR is known as "Dead Bird." The following lessons are representative of the group. In these lessons, the eye-hand connection, which is part of the reflex, is incorporated as well.

> *AY 041: Basic Bending – (Reel 3/4/4)*
> *AM 1 – Week 2 – June 17 AM1: Seated*
> *and Twist Left (part 1) ["Dead Bird"]*
> *AY 420: In Sitting – Twisting With*
> *the Eyes – (Reel 27/2/4)*

The base position in these lessons is side sitting, leaning on one hand, holding the other arm lifted in front of the face with the hand hanging down and the eyes fixed on the hand.

In the string of movements, the upper part of the body turns to one side, at first as one unit, followed by separating and differentiating the turning movements of the trunk, the shoulders, the head, and the eyes. The sequence is repeated alternating the order of the moving parts, and to both sides.

The lessons flag the extension of the body moving away from its center and back toward it, the differentiation between the various parts of the upper body, and the hand-eyes connection, which are all features of the reflex.

Tonic labyrinthine reflex (TLR)

The tonic labyrinthine reflex activates the postural dynamics that assist the infant to get up from the floor and to control the body against gravity. This reflex is responsible for the development of postural stability and head control; it helps to develop the vestibular system and prepares the infant for further motor development.

The reflex has two components: in the forward TLR, as the head bends forward, the whole body, arms, legs, and torso, curl inward in the characteristic fetal position. In the backward TLR, as the head bends backward, the whole body, arms, legs, and torso straighten and extend.

This reflex teaches the infant to straighten out from the fetal position. The reflex helps to develop the muscles needed to manage the weight of the head and the limbs and to align the head with the rest of the body for balance and visual tracking, which is necessary to focus and learning. When this reflex remains partially active and not fully integrated, the person may have poor posture and poor spatial orientation. For the participant, this lesson can be very effective in reinforcing those same features and the carriage of the head.

AY 076: Slow Lifting; On the Stomach – (Reel 6/2/5)
When lying face down and lifting the head, the infant is sensitized to his/her body pressing against the floor. This interaction teaches the infant to gain control under the force of gravity, which is one of the outcomes of the TLR. This schema is reproduced in this lesson.

The importance of lifting the head we saw in chapter 5 in lesson AY 057. Here, the head is lifted in conjunction with other parts of the body, helping to erect the spine and extend the body.

Lying face down, a sequence follows of the smallest possible lifting of the head, the arms, and the legs. The movements are made in different arrangements, such as each limb or the head alone, and in pairs combining head and arms, arms and legs, and head and legs. Attention is on the floor and on the parts of the body that press against it during the lifting, thereby marking the pull of gravity and refining the counterforce deployed against it. The lesson is effective in improving balance and posture.

AY 058: Transferring Support While On the Stomach –
(Reel 4/4/3)
This lesson continues the main movements of the last one, but this time with full and large movements, rather than slight and soft. The lesson reproduces the extension and flexion active in the reflex.

Lying face down, with the body extended, and with the arms, the head, and the legs raised, rocking the body back and forth from each hip joint to the opposite arm-pit, the ground support of the body is sensed travelling in a diagonal line. Again, with legs, arms, and head raised, support is transferred forward and backward between the chest and inflated belly. In another variation in the same position, the support is transferred by pressing the area in an approximate circle around the stomach, as in a clock traveling through all the numbers. The movement is repeated lying face up, holding the soles with the hands, flexing the body, and rocking on a small circle of support on the curved back.

AY 222: On the Abdomen, a Hand Lifting the Head –
(Reel 16/1/1)

In this lesson, much as in the two lessons above, the back flexes and extends while the chest softens. The string of movements includes lying face down, the head turned to the side lying on the hands one on top of the other, the hand under the head lifting it, contracting the back. This movement is also done with the knee bent and foot raised with the sole facing the ceiling, and turning the eyes to see the heel. In a variation, also lying face down, the knee is bent and the foot raised toward the ceiling, and the hand on the same side takes hold of the ankle. Partially straightening the leg toward the floor lifts the head and shoulder and "draws" the back like a bow.

Symmetrical tonic neck reflex (STNR)

The symmetrical tonic neck reflex, also known as the crawling reflex, consists of two phases: flexion (inward movement) and extension (outward movement). When the child is positioned on hands and knees, flexion or lowering of the head causes the arms to bend and the legs to extend. When the neck is extended and the head raised, the arms extend and the legs bend. When the head is lowered, the arms bend and the legs extend. Whereas the ATNR divides the body in half vertically, and the TLR divides the body between back and front, the STNR divides the body in half horizontally—the upper and lower body.

This reflex, developed after the ATNR, educates the infant to defy gravity on hands and knees and helps to raise and control the head for far-distance focusing, which is a stepping stone to advance to the crawling phase.

The reflex emerges between 6 and 9 months of life and should be integrated by 12 months. If this reflex remains active, the infant's crawling will be affected. The proper integration of the STNR is very important in visual development as well, since the infant gets the experience of visually tracking the hands as they move forward in space, which helps to develop the ability of the eyes to cross the midline when tracking. The sense of balance, the perception of space and depth, as well as eye-hand coordination are closely tied to the appropriate integration of the STNR.[i] The following lessons echo all these features, refreshing posture, the sense of balance, and space perception in the participant.

---

[i] Some of the symptoms that indicate a deficient integration of the STNR are: poor eye-hand coordination, difficulty adjusting binocular vision from distance to near, and poor balance. See Berne 2006.

AY 057: Lifting the Head on All Fours – (Reel 4/4/2)

This lesson, which we saw in chapter 5 in relation to crawling, replicates the STNR with all its elements. It includes the flexion and extension movements while standing on the knees and hands, as well as the lowering of the head while bending the arms and extending the legs. The lesson sharpens the ability to arch the spine and the movement of the eyes within the field of sight.

Other lessons that reproduce some features of the reflex and improve the ability to arch the spine are the following two:

AY 370: Lifting the Head – (Reel 24/3/9)

The lesson reproduces the outward movement of the reflex. Lying face down, with an ear on the back of one hand, and with a knee bent sideways, the head is lifted with the hand's help. The back is arched, further helped by combining several movements of the legs, such as raising the extended leg, with the lifting of the head supported by the hand. The movements lengthen the front of the spine, making the arching smoother and softening the chest.

AY 177: Making the Spine Flexible and Integrating it – (Reel 13/1/1)

This lesson lengthens the spine by flexing and extending the back. Lying face up, the pelvis is raised, slowly, gradually, vertebra by vertebra, arching the back and elongating the spine from the coccyx upward. At the other end of the body, the head is lifted by the two hands with interlaced fingers, flexing the upper spine until it meets the arched lower spine. From here, a wavelike movement travels from the bottom of the spine to the head and back, extending and flexing the back of the body, which lengthens the spine and increases flexibility. The flexion and extension of the back is also done by raising and lowering the head on knees and hands, and on knees and forearms.

Moro reflex

The Moro reflex, sometimes called the infant startle reflex, is an involuntary protective motor response against sudden loss of support, a disruption of body balance, or an extremely unexpected stimulus such as sudden bright light, loud noise, or temperature change. When this happens, the hands open, and the arms and legs are briskly extended away from the body and to the sides, then drawn together as if in an embrace as the hands close.

The reflex is fully developed at 38 weeks of fetal life, and it gradually disappears by the age of 3–6 months. If it remains active It may signal chronic, nonprogressive motor disabilities of cerebral origin. The extension and flexion of arms and legs prepare the infant to roll. The following lesson reproduces the sequence of movements.

AY 313: Rolling at the Rate of Stretching and Bending – (Reel 21/4/1)

This lesson, examined in the previous chapter, comprises the basic movements of the Moro reflex, which are extension and flexion of the body, the opening of the arms and legs, and the movement of the head backward and the stomach forward.

The reflexes examined here are not the only primitive and early life reflexes. These, however, are the basis of motor development that goes from rolling to standing up and walking. Among other primitive reflexes reproduced in some lessons, and worth mentioning, is the palmar reflex. This reflex is the automatic flexing of fingers to grab an object, activated by a mechanical stimulus to the palm. It is present in a newborn, and has been observed already in the fetal period when the infant grasps the umbilical cord. It is the basis for fine motor skills. In the Amherst course we find a series of lessons reproducing the reflex, aiming to enliven dormant brain maps of those movements.[i]

Primitive and early life reflexes are features encoded genetically in the organism that trigger involuntary movements, and are the basis of motor development. When the movements become voluntary and the infant learns to roll, stand, and walk, the reflexes are not removed from the organism's memory. They have been inherited from the ancestors, and are kept by every person for further transmission. Their template remains part of the organism, though

---

[i] AM 2 – Week 1 – June 10 PM2: "On Back Flexing Torso/Bell Crawl."

AM 2 – Week 1 – June 11 AM1: "Swimming Crawl/Bell Hand, Think Toes."

AM 2 – Week 1 – June 11 AM2: "Swimming Crawl/Bell Hand, Think Toes (cont'd)."

it is relegated to another sphere of the brain: using Damasio's words, "we let them go underground, into the roomy basement of our minds."[i]

The process of transformation that the Feldenkrais Method activates brings to somatic awareness the roots of the movements of the body. The person does not become conscious of the reflex, but the body, the organism that harbors the codes, recognizes itself, so to speak. By going to the roots of the movements, the method makes it possible for the body to recall and, eventually, to reframe and reset the moments of inception of the movements, and in doing so, the self-image.

---

[i] Damasio 2010, p. 275

7

Habits and Their Renewal:
Doing the Same Action Differently

The third path for self-transformation that the Feldenkrais Method follows, bringing to the surface nonconscious patterns deep-rooted in the original sensorimotor schema and the nervous system, is the restructuring of habitual movements.

Habits, in general, regulate significant functions and capacities of the body's movements and of the character of the person. Habits encompass a great variety of acts and practices, including walking, sitting, carrying loads, driving, and the work that people do for a living. Also "the reaction of the nervous system to the pull of gravity is a habit," as Feldenkrais affirms.[i] Other habits are the practices of everyday life, such as how people cook and eat, the music they listen to, their sleeping practices, what people do in their free time, and the like. All these arrangements and body movements are part of habitual behavior and are fundamental in shaping the self-image.

---

[i] *Embodied Wisdom*, p. 35.

In essence, habits are very important in people's lives, since they contribute to smoother functioning, without the need to expend much thought, effort, or stress in regular, everyday doings. Habits economize the body's energy and allow people to engage in other activities while simultaneously undertaking routine tasks. They are essential in the management of life.[i]

And yet, these advantages can turn into disadvantages, and adaptations to the conditions of life that could have been beneficial at one time can become detrimental. There may be different reasons for this; one is that the functionality of a habit has wasted away, like the loss of a skill. Another reason is that habitual movements can become mechanical or even compulsive, and can cause tensions and pain. In this situation, one's behavior, actions, and movements may be negatively affected.[ii]

Under these circumstances, habits can block the possibility of reflection and awareness of one's own movements and behavior, to the point of draining every drop of creativity out of those practices and actions. As such, habits can obstruct the acquisition of new and different forms of behavior and bodily expression, thereby impeding attunement to changing situations in life.

After habits have taken shape, their structure and the chain of steps that forge the movement are not forgotten, but rather archived below the threshold of consciousness. They are deeply wired behaviors, stored as neurological maps that allow the brain to follow the

---

[i] See Caruana and Testa 2020. For an analysis of the relation between habits and the self, see Wagner et al. 2014.

[ii] See *The Potent Self: A Study of Spontaneity and Compulsion*, chap. 2.

same route without having to think, thus freeing it to engage in other activities.

The lessons of the Feldenkrais Method are vehicles to access and revise those maps. The aim is to travel the original paths and patterns and, at the same time, to disrupt them by opening other routes for the movements. The purpose is to reset the most ingrained habits and to renew those movements by generating more-efficient modes of action. This is not a simple process, since, as Feldenkrais asserts, "our nervous system is so constructed that habits are preserved and seek to perpetuate themselves." The way to achieve it is "to pay close attention to every improvement and to assimilate it after every series of movements."[i]

The modus operandi of the Feldenkrais Method is, indeed, to deconstruct actions into their basic components and reassemble them anew with a more inclusive integration of the body parts. The action is then redesigned. Examples of this strategy we saw above in chapter 5, "Rolling to sit," where the lessons disassemble the act of sitting up to its components and show how, by joining into the movement the elbows, the shoulders, and the head, an organized skeletal system can sit effortlessly. Also, in the "Dead Bird" lessons (chapter 6), where a simple habitual movement such as turning the head is transformed by incorporating into the movement the eyes, the thorax, the shoulders, the pelvis, and the knees. By highlighting non-habitual movements and disrupting routine patterns, the Feldenkrais Method offers more-comfortable alternative pathways for the same actions.

---

[i] *Awareness Through Movement*, p.127.

What is significant to notice is that the Feldenkrais Method teaches both a different way to do the same action and the fact that there *are* different ways of doing it. The aim is double: to recreate the self-image by changing habitual movements, and to heighten awareness of the possibility of self-change.

Non-habitual movements – The Lessons

Non-habitual movements are of utmost importance in the Feldenkrais Method, opening up fresh possibilities for posture and action. Practicing non-habitual movements awakens awareness of the skeleton's ductility and of different ways to organize the movements, and intervenes in the way the self-image is experienced.

We can distinguish three different kinds of non-habitual movements. One, found in most if not all of the lessons, is movements that have not been previously experienced or that are very unusual, such as lying on the back and lengthening the arms by pushing the floor with one foot (AY 345); sitting and turning the shoulders and the head in one direction, while turning the eyes in the other direction (AY 420); and crawling crossing one leg through in front of the other (E 27/Es 25, AY 502). Here I examine another category, those that combine everyday habitual movements with non-habitual movements. A third kind of non-habitual movements is the reproduction of the chain of motor development in reverse (I will visit this in chapter 8).

I have chosen lessons with different combinations of non-habitual standing and walking. Their aim is to improve acture in walking by practicing standing and walking in non-usual ways, and by incorporating into the movement parts of the body that are usually inactive or sensorially mute in that specific action.

Having correct posture in standing and walking was a theme of personal interest to Feldenkrais, as he had suffered from painful knee problems.[i] Feldenkrais's thorough exploration of the theme can be appreciated in the rich repertoire of modes of standing and walking.

Non-habitual standing

AY 078: Standing – (Reel 6/3/2)

The objective of this lesson is to improve standing and prepare for walking. It is an asymmetric lesson that guides the right foot to stand and shows the difference of a foot that is better organized from one that is less so— the left foot. Lifting only the right foot in most of the movements brings the sense of balance into attention.

The reference movement is standing on one leg, loosening the other knee, and lifting that foot from the floor. Different movements of the arms and hands alternate, such as caressing the leg to reach the knee and the foot while lifting the knee toward the chest, first with one hand, then in various combinations of the two hands. The movements help to organize the hips, arms, shoulder girdle, and legs for standing. The movements are repeated lying face up.

AY 283: Continuation on One Leg – (Reel 19/4/3)

This lesson seeks to improve standing and walking by experiencing a shift of the weight completely onto one

---

[i] On the importance of how Feldenkrais handled his knee problem, and its relation to the method, see Reese 2015, chaps. 2, 4, and 5.

heel to free the other leg and with the back erect but round, which are two main features of integrated walking.

The reference position and movements are standing and pivoting one heel outward while simultaneously lifting the other foot from the floor. The organization of the standing position on one leg stimulates the sense of balance. Attention during the lesson is on breathing, on the freedom of the neck, and on the gaze.

AY 484: In Standing – Turning With the Eyes – (Reel 31/3/3)

This lesson animates the proprioceptive sense and the shift of weight from one foot to the other.

In standing, the main movements are twisting the head and shoulders to look over the shoulder. The twisting is done by lifting the foot slightly and turning the heel outward, transferring the weight to the turning foot. The direction of the eyes is differentiated from and then reintegrated with the head and torso. The movement develops into a free turning back and forth, with arms swinging, and into a 360° spin.

AY 289: Standing on One Leg With Movements – (Reel 20/2/1)

The non-habitual movements in this lesson aim to improve standing by incorporating parts of the body that are usually not purposely active in habitual standing.

The movements, in standing, include hanging one arm to the side, and letting the weight of the arm lift the opposite leg and foot from the floor; with the same arm reaching over the head and taking hold of the opposite temple, bending and leaning to the side lifts the opposite foot from the floor. In all the movements it is the weight of the moving parts that acts as a lever on the foot, lifting it from the floor. The movements activate the sense of balance and facilitate a suppler standing posture.

Non-habitual walking

AY 501: Introduction to Walking – (Reel 33/1/1)

The lesson, reviewed above (chapter 5), seeks to improve acture in walking by practicing non-habitual walking.

Different forms of non-habitual walking are experimented with, such as walking while taking one hip back and forward, then the other; walking with the arms close to the body without moving them; walking while bringing one ear close to the shoulder, and then the other. All these non-habitual movements activate parts of the body and the skeletal schema that usually are not actively and deliberately set in motion when walking.

AY 502: Walking and Crawling – (Reel 33/1/2)

With this lesson, also reviewed above, we can fully appreciate how experimenting with non-habitual movements revitalizes habitual movements—how non-habitual variants of an everyday movement, such as walking, can restore stability to posture and gait, making them more balanced and better organized.

The lesson combines habitual with non-habitual walking as well as habitual with non-habitual crawling on all fours, on the stomach, and on the back. These forms of crawling antecede bipedalism in human beings, and the habitual/non-habitual experimentation in this lesson goes to the very origins of walking.

AY 503: Hopping and Arms – (Reel 33/1/3)

This lesson experiments with a whole variety of non-habitual movements of legs, arms, shoulders, hips, and head while walking. The movements seek to incorporate parts of the body that are not intentionally actuated in habitual walking, to facilitate suppleness of acture.

The movements include walking with arms and legs alternating between the habitual and non-habitual synchronies; bringing the hips and shoulders to move in sync but in opposite directions, such as moving the right shoulder forward while the right hip goes backward; hopping with extended hands above the head, and opening them in unison with the legs, then opening the hands when the legs come close to each other (like a gentle hopping version of "jumping jacks"). Also included is walking sideways and raising the hands with each sidestep, then reversing the combination—lowering the hands with each sidestep and raising them when legs scissor together.

AY 504: Continuation and Return – (Reel 33/1/4)

This lesson invents absurd and ingenious non-habitual forms of walking, and shows how movements of the upper part of the body change the way we walk. Some of the movements are: walking hunched, with the back bowed forward and the arms hanging, crouching and bending as if rolling a ball with the hand along the floor (as the ball grows smaller, the curve of the back gets larger); putting the arms behind the back and holding each forearm or elbow with the other hand, sliding the elbows to one side and tilting the head to the opposite side with each step. The lesson explores stability and balance in the different configurations, disrupting and refreshing habitual walking.

AY 138: Walking on the Heels – (Reel 10/2/4)

Alternating between habitual and non-habitual walking in different forms, this lesson seeks to make smoother and more efficient the pattern of moving all the limbs while walking. The different forms include raising the toes and walking on the heels only, and the opposite, walking on the toes by raising the heels. Another form is hopping on the heels, and then hopping on the toes. There is also walking on the heels with tiny steps forward, to the right, backward, and to the left—in a square.

8

How Do We Know When a
Movement Has Been Mastered?

The answer to this important question is simple: when you can do the movement backward. Starting from the end of a movement and finalizing it at what is usually the beginning proves that the movement has been learned and acquired. In Feldenkrais's words: "The main feature of correct acture or posture in all … voluntary actions is reversibility."[i]

More than the capacity to do the movement starting from the end, reversibility is the capacity to stop a movement at any point and then go in any direction with a minimum of hesitation. The movement is fully mastered when "At every instant or stage of a correct act, it can be stopped, withheld from continuing, or reversed without any preliminary change of attitude and without effort."[ii]

In sum, reversibility is the ability to move in any direction with a minimum of vacillation or preparation, by pivoting and changing

---

[i] *The Potent Self,* p. 113.
[ii] Ibid.

direction while shifting the weight effortlessly. This means that when standing, sitting, or walking, moving forward or backward are equally available movements. The quality of preparedness to move anywhere is an ideal state of affairs that represents the highest level of physical organization.

Doing them backward – The Lessons

Numerous lessons contain elements of reversibility, such as when an arm initiates the movement of a leg by pulling the knee, and then the knee initiates the same or opposite movement by pulling the arm; or when movements are done in one direction and then in the opposite direction. In this chapter, I present lessons that reproduce the movements of the chain of motor development done in reverse order.

Sitting to lying

AY 326: Sitting – Lying – (Reel 22/3/2)

This lesson reverses the main movements of AY 327 (chapter 5), by bringing the body from the sitting position to lying face up.

Sitting with extended, spread legs and leaning to the side, the elbow comes to the floor, and the opposite leg and sit bone lift from the floor. The movement is repeated with the legs in the same position but holding them with the hands under the knees, which, together with the weight of the head and the upper body tilting onto one elbow, lifts the opposite leg and sit bone from the floor. Then, lifting both legs in the air while balancing on the buttocks, expanding the abdomen forward, then toward one leg and then the other; arching and curving the back, and rolling the support around the sit bones in a circle, the body comfortably comes to lie on the back, and then up to sitting again.

Sitting to rolling

AY 417: Preparation for Rolling to Sitting – (Reel 27/2/1)
E 35: Initiation in Rolling/Es 33: Introduction to Rolling
These two almost identical lessons are preparations for rolling to sitting by going from sitting to rolling, which inverts the natural process of learning how to sit up. It is "a starting from the end." These lessons reverse the main movements of lesson AY 067 (chapter 5).

From the sitting position, with the legs bent, soles of the feet together, and each hand holding the corresponding ankle, a slow rocking to the side brings the elbow close to the floor, and the opposite leg rises. Directing the elbow in front of the knee on the floor until it touches slightly brings the whole body, leaning-turning, in the direction of the floor. Then, in the same position, holding the opposite leg by the ankle, and moving the foot apart from the other foot and away from the body, back and forth, the knee of the moving leg comes toward the body when the foot moves away, and moves away from the body when the foot comes back and the soles again touch.

These oscillatory and hyperbolic movements, combined with the body leaning to the other side and the elbow touching the floor, organize the body for half rolling. The knee moving away from the body works as a lever for full rolling, and brings the body back to the sitting position. In the end, the momentum generates a circular movement that goes from sitting to rolling to sitting uninterruptedly.

Crawling to sitting

E 27: Primitive Locomotion: Coordinating the Locomotive Joints/Es 25: Crawling, on Knees

Crawling comes after the infant has mastered sitting up. In this lesson (examined above, chapter 5), the movements are reversed as a means to refine their integration.

The string of movements proceeds from standing on hands and knees to sitting on the heels, and then crawling in a non-habitual way. Crawling is done by crossing one leg through in front of the other, or sliding it back behind the other. The crawling is built step by step, sliding and crossing a leg between the opposite hand and knee, and raising and lowering the head.

Standing to sitting

AY 145: From Sitting to Standing While Turning – (Reel 10/4/3)

The lesson brings the participant from sitting to standing and back to sitting, following the same path.

The reference position is sitting with the soles together and arms held in front in a large circle like an embrace, eyes on the point where the fingertips touch. Turning the shoulders, arms, pelvis, and head together as one from side to side, and shifting the weight from sit bone to sit bone, the movement develops into a swing that enables a natural rise to standing on the knees, which in turn grows to a standing position after bringing one foot forward to stand on the floor.

After this sequence, movements are done in reverse, from the standing position placing one hand on the floor and turning the pelvis around 180 degrees as it comes down to sit cross-legged on the floor. It is then easier to rise to standing from the initial position of sitting with the soles together and the arms "hugging" in front.

Walking and standing

AY 354: Walking Backward – (Reel 24/2/1)

This lesson shows how to organize the body to walk backward. The sequence starts in standing, holding to a chair to keep balance, lifting one heel, then lowering the heel and standing on both legs without putting any weight into the heel. The action is repeated with one foot behind, on the toes, then lowering the heel, again weightlessly. This is possible by letting the hip and hip joint move backward and the base of the skull and the head lift upward and forward. It is the longitude of the spine that increases, freeing the heel from carrying weight. This set-up of movements lays the groundwork for walking backward.

Walking backward is explored in different ways, such as with elbows lifted and spread to the sides with the arms raised and lowered. Attention is on the connection and the distance between the heel, the hip joint, and the base of the skull.

9

Transformation as Transference

The term *transference* was made popular by Sigmund Freud, as the name for a key component in his psychoanalytic theory and practice. The term refers to the unconscious redirection of the feelings a person (the psychoanalytic patient) has about a second person (usually an important figure from early life—parent, grandparent, sibling) to a third person (the psychoanalyst), affording a chance for those feelings to be brought into awareness.

Feldenkrais was well acquainted with and valued Freud's theory, and used the term in his writings and lessons, but not in its psychoanalytic sense.[i] Feldenkrais was influenced by the works of Schilder and the psychologist Émile Coué, who, working along different lines, gave an embodied twist to the Freudian term, having experimented and

---

[i] For Feldenkrais's use of the term "transference" see the Esalen, San Francisco, and Amherst seminars, and *The Potent Self: A Study of Spontaneity and Compulsion.*

theorized on the transference of feelings and sensations from the mind to the body, and on the effects of such processes on the nervous tissue.[i]

Feldenkrais goes deeper, to the sensorimotor level, and adopts the idea of redirecting a sensation or feeling, but neither from a person to another person nor from the mind to the body, but rather from one part of the body to another. He had learned from the pathophysiologist Alekseĭ Speransky that "the body reacts physiologically almost as a fundamentally new entity after certain irritations of the nervous tissue,"[ii] which explains how functionality can be transferred from a part of the body to another part. The idea is, indeed, to redirect the functionality of one part of the body to another part that is less functionally organized, knowing that this is aided by the flow of information in the nervous system.

In the Esalen workshop, Feldenkrais gave a pair of lessons that epitomize what he means by transference as a means for transformation.

> ### E 23: Left Shoulder Differentiation and Reintegration Into the Self-Image/Es 22: Left Shoulder, Lying on Side
> This is an asymmetric lesson that focuses on the range of motion in different directions of the left shoulder. While lying on the right side, the sequence includes moving the shoulder forward and backward, up (toward the left ear) and down (toward the hip), and in circles, as well as discerning how the ribs, the pelvis, the legs, the arms, and the head can participate in articulating the

---

[i] On the influence of Schilder on Feldenkrais, see the "Foreword" to *Body and Mature Behavior* by Carl Ginsburg. On Coué and Feldenkrais see chapter 11.

[ii] *Body and Mature Behavior*, 6. On Speransky and Feldenkrais, see Reese 2015, chap. 5.

reach of the shoulder and shoulder blade. The movement becomes clearer, easier, and freer after the constraints on those other parts are removed, and by involving the whole of the body in the movements. This lesson provides full control and freedom of movement to the left shoulder in all directions.

The lesson that followed this one in the Esalen seminar was a continuation of the former, aiming at expanding and spreading the freedom, organization, and integration achieved in the left shoulder to the rest of the body.[i] The lesson uses the functionally integrated left shoulder as an axis of movements done with other parts of the body.

Feldenkrais introduces the lesson as follows:

> We are going to integrate our "good" shoulder into our body's other movements. Our good shoulder will demand improvements of the neck, of the spine, of the rest of the body. It demands that we become nimbler, simpler, stronger, more flexible. Because of the shoulder's improvement, it wants to move better, and demands that the rest of the body improve also.[ii]

I should underscore that the transfer of the functionality of the organized shoulder is not limited to freedom and clarity of movement, but also extends to the sensorial layer, as Feldenkrais explains:

---

[i] E 24: "Raising the Entire Self to Function With a Live Shoulder"/
  Es 23: "Integrating Whole Body With the Improved Shoulder from Lesson 22."
[ii] *Esalen 1972 Workshop*, p. 143.

> In the previous lesson we differentiated the left shoulder. The problem is to transfer that sensation to the other shoulder; in fact, to the whole body—to thinking, to feeling.[i]

Here we find another clue to answer the question raised in chapter 3: Where to start a Functional Integration (FI) lesson? The idea here is to look for the part of the body or the articulation that moves most freely and to expand that quality to other parts of the body that feel obstructed. Having found that place, the suggestion is to follow the flow of movement until it does not flow, then stop and look for ways to release the obstruction. This can be by looking for other chains of movements that might meet the obstructed place in a different way, or by any other way that the practitioner deems appropriate. Indeed, as a method of change and transformation, the Feldenkrais Method aims to spread the freedom of movement of the more integrated parts and articulations of the body to the less integrated, and indeed to our consciousness and our self-image as a whole.

---

[i] Ibid.

PART THREE

SENSING THE BODY FROM WITHIN

10

Body Meditation

Long-lasting modifications of the functional integration of the body movements and posture, and the attuning of the body-self-image and self-change, are the result of a regular and suitable practice that goes hand in hand with somatic awareness. The Feldenkrais Method uses two main devices to awaken awareness and the sensorial consciousness of the body, which are body meditation and imagination.

Body meditation, in its different forms, relaxes, slows the heartbeat, decreases respiratory rate, and restores energy. It ultimately brings balance between the sympathetic and parasympathetic nervous system and is a health-enhancing procedure. In the Feldenkrais Method, body meditation serves to strengthen and amplify somatic awareness as well.

The main meditational tool of the Feldenkrais Method is *scanning*. It is noticeable that during the last decades scanning of the body has become a popular practice in the Western world for meditative purposes. The practice consists, mainly, of a body scan that can be performed while lying down, sitting, or in other positions. The idea is to relax the muscles and bring close attention to the body and to both "loud" and subtle sensations noticed as the person does a mental scan from heel to head and back. Today this technique is used to help find stability of spirit and temperament, and to cultivate mindfulness.

This practice is identical to what Feldenkrais used more than fifty years ago, undoubtedly inspired by other cultural and religious sources. In addition to scanning, the Feldenkrais Method has other forms of body meditation developed into full lessons. Worth mentioning are breathing and bowing-praying lessons. What characterizes the meditative lessons of the method is the combination of simple, soft, slow, sensitized movements with the power of imagination.

The Lessons

Scanning

Scanning is one of the most important meditative ingredients the Feldenkrais Method uses to enliven and stimulate awareness. Most lessons begin with a partial or full scan of the body, and in all the lessons, scanning recurs in a short form several times during pauses, as well as at the end. Usually the scan brings attention to the parts of the body that the lesson is focused on. Other lessons are specifically directed to the meditative aspect of scanning, which they develop fully.

The lesson "Scanning: General Remarks" (E 2) is representative of this distinctive form of body meditation. We have already examined this lesson above (in chapter 2), concerning the five cardinal lines that form the self-image. There, I called attention to the way awareness of the line of the spine is brightened by scanning with the aid of imagination, using two imaginary fingers to press along the spine. Other body meditation lessons mentioned in that same chapter are "Repose (this is your skeleton),"[i] where scanning is done through the small bones of the body, from fingers to toes via ankles, knees, and shoulders; and "Simpler" (AY 339), where awareness is raised by gently moving while sensing and imagining the dimensions of and distances between the legs, arms, hip joints, and shoulders.

There are other lessons that have scanning as their major theme, and where we can appreciate its power to highlight parts of the body that are partially or fully mute. One of them is the following.

AY 496: The Face – (Reel 32/3/2)

In this lesson, the right side of the face is scanned thoroughly, including all of its parts, such as nose, ears, eyes, chin, palate, and forehead. The participant is guided both to touch and to scan without hands (as well as to warm with imagined sun rays) the surface of the different parts of the face, its inside, and its interface with the immediately surrounding space. The scanning also attends to the geometrical relations between the different parts of the face, such as the length of the nose and the line between the ear and the eye, as well as the angle of the jaw. The relation of the face to the neck, the torso, and the right leg is touched on. As a one-sided lesson, this highlights the difference that awareness brings to any part of the self-image.

---

[i] Reel 9/3/2, this lesson is not included in the Alexander Yanai Collections.

Other lessons that scan parts of the face in different ways are "The Eyeball Lesson,"[i] which explores the eyeballs, their size, weight, and contours, including the sockets; and "Palate, Mouth, and Teeth,"[ii] which does the same with the internal space of the palate and teeth, helped by the tongue and the imagination.

Breathing

Breathing is a vital function, and the foundation of movement, health, and well-being. Breathing affects the entire body and has a significant role in postural stability and mobility of the trunk and spine. Mindful breathing is a meditative practice of physical and emotional benefits, such as reduction of stress, relaxation, and preventing anxiety.[iii]

In the Feldenkrais Method, breathing is underscored in all of the lessons. To maintain regular breathing while making the movements is the baseline teaching; it is a common habit to hold the breath while concentrating or venturing something new, and Feldenkrais Method lessons draw attention to this habit, which can inhibit learning. But there are also full lessons with breathing as the main theme, and some of these make conscious changes to spontaneous breathing to highlight aspects of the process. These lessons explore the rhythm and flow of the air filling the lungs, and what happens to and in the body when breathing: how, when air flows through the lungs, it raises and lowers the abdomen, the chest, and the diaphragm, and how the

---

[i] AY 165 – (Reel 12/2/1).

[ii] AY 023 – (Reel 2/3/5).

[iii] For scientific publications on mindful breathing, a search with Google Scholar gives more than 75,000 sources of professional journals and books. Accessed May 10. 2022.

lungs and thorax shrink when the air is exhaled. These air experimentations make the body present from the inside.

AY 017: Breathing – (Reel 2/2/2)
AY 021: Contracting the Abdomen While Exhaling –
(Reel 2/3/2)

These lessons instruct how breathing is done, by sensing how the abdomen contracts when exhaling in various positions and orientations of the body, such as lying facing up, face down, on the side, and on all fours. Attention is paid to the movements of the thorax, the ribs, the arms, and the head during breathing. AY 017 is mainly a lecture on the theme, guiding the participants to become aware of formerly unconscious restrictions on the full potential of breathing.

AY 172: Stopping the Breath – (Reel 12/3/5)

With gentle movements and in a variety of positions, this lesson guides the participants to increase their sensitivity and awareness of the air going into and out of the lungs.

Stopping the breath, both in inhalation and exhalation, explores the transition from one to the other and the movements of different parts of the body, such as the abdomen, chest, shoulder blades, and diaphragm. The breathing movements are experimented with lying face down with the arms forward above the head; on the back with knees bent; sitting with the soles together; and on the stomach, lifting elbows and head from the floor. Changing pressure on the floor brings more awareness to the parts of the body that move in breathing and the symmetry or asymmetry of the two sides. According to Feldenkrais, in the process of stopping inhaling and exhaling, "the system itself recalibrates the atlas and axis," which facilitates correcting posture and the carriage of the head.

ATM Lesson 4: Differentiation of Parts and Functions in Breathing

This lesson covers different functions, rhythms, and movements of breathing. The major themes are the change in volume of the chest when breathing; the movements and volume of the lower abdomen; seesaw movements of the diaphragm; and the curvature of the spine when breathing. The relation between posture and breathing is the central theme of this lesson. The idea is "that breathing becomes easier and more rhythmical when the body is held erect without any conscious effort, that is, when its entire weight is supported by the skeletal structure."[i]

Bowing–Praying

Bowing is both a physical and a spiritual, meditative action. Considering the anatomic functionality of bowing, the focus is on the cervical spine, whose primary function is to provide support for the skull while still allowing for movement. It is the most flexible part of the spine,

---

[i] *Awareness Through Movement*, p. 100.

enabling large movements of the head to scan the surroundings. Most of the sensory inputs that the human being receives occur at the head; thus, a correct and dynamic head-neck connection is crucial for movement and survival.

Bending and lifting the head and neck continuously and gently with regular breathing, relaxed by leaving aside all effort and tension of the muscles, is a quintessential meditative practice. Certainly, the meditative power of bowing is seen through many different lenses, embodying human acts rich with meaning. Bowing is a human practice with a long tradition in the cultural, religious, and spiritual spheres of life. The movement itself is seen as the enactment and manifestation of the force of gravity, connecting the high and the low, the earth with the zenith. In religious practices, it is an integral part of the act of praying. As a body gesture, particularly in Eastern cultures, it conveys awe, humbleness, respect toward the other person, the divinity and its teachings.

The series of lessons that have bowing and praying as a main theme seek to integrate the simple movement of bowing with the rest of the body, and improve the flexibility and smooth functioning of the head-neck ensemble. The meditative, spiritual aspect, however, does not go unnoticed.

AY 046: Lowering the Head – (Reel 4/1/4)
AY 050: Lowering the Head – (Reel 4/2/4)

Gently lowering and raising the head activates the cervical vertebrae one by one, expanding the space between each adjacent two of them, elongating the spine, and adding flexibility to the movements of the head. These lessons seek to soften the movement of the head when lowering it by attending to the other places in the body where the movement resonates.

In AY 046, attention while lowering the head goes to the distance and relations between the ear and the knee, the eye and the ear, and the changes felt while bowing. Other movements seeking to enact flexibility and soften the cervical spine are lowering the head and swinging it slowly from side to side in a pendulum trajectory, activating the shoulders. The pendulum movements are also done with the head back and the face towards the ceiling and standing on one knee and one foot, attending to the balance of the body. AY 050 also involves spinal flexion and extension in several different positions, both symmetric and asymmetric. Positions include sitting, on all fours, kneeling, sphinx, and semi-reclined. Bowing is done, as well, in half-sitting/half-lying face up with shoulders and head raised on the elbows and forearms, and on hands and knees.

AY 363: Prayer – (Reel 24/3/2)
AM 1 – Week 7 – July 24 AM1: Morning Prayer

In these lessons the bowing movement combines with the palm-to-palm praying-hands gesture. In the two similar lessons, the initial movements are, in sitting, lowering and raising the head and the praying hands together without altering the distance between them. The movements are also done separately, only with the hands, and only with the head; turning to each side with the head and hands together, and then

> alternating the hands and the head to opposite sides.
> The movements are repeated on the knees, noting the
> connection between the movements of the head and of
> the pelvis.

With these lessons, and the series of lessons that have bowing or praying as a theme, Feldenkrais remits us to an historic human practice, an ancient ritual, expressed in specific body movements: a practice, similar in different and diverse religions, embodied in a gesture that incorporates movements of the head, the hands, and the knees. The palm-to-palm hands position is a prayer gesture ubiquitous in Christianity, and in Hindu and Buddhist traditions it is a sign of greeting, respect, and veneration. The lessons explore body movements that are part of old traditions, and wrapped in spiritual and religious feelings.[i]

In *Morning Prayer*, Feldenkrais speaks about the inherent relationship of those movements to religious beliefs and to blessing. As an example, he points to the movements and gestures of the Pope making the sign of the cross and blessing as expressions of the deep belief and devotion of the addresser transmitted to the addressees. For Feldenkrais the act of praying, its movements and history, go

---

[i] During the time that Feldenkrais was learning and teaching judo and ju-jitsu in France, he had extensive contact with Eastern tradition and practices. All the more so, he integrated the theme of the *tanden* (or *dantian*, or *hara*), a concept used to describe a major source of body energy in some of the internal and external martial arts, in several lessons, such as AY 351: "Swinging the Legs on the Side" – (Reel 24/1/5), and AY 359: "Tanden with Bending the Knees" – (Reel 24/2/6). See the introductions by Michael Brousse, Dennis Leri, and Moti Nativ to *Higher Judo*. For the Buddhist antecedents of body scan meditation, see Anālayo 2020.

deep into the realms of the non- or unconscious. In this regard he considered prayer a form of autosuggestion, known to our ancestors for generations.[i]

---

[i] See Feldenkrais's view on prayer as a religious practice in "Last in deed, first in thought," in *Thinking and Doing*. More on this theme in Part Four.

11

Imagination

Imagination is a powerful tool that the Feldenkrais Method uses to enhance awareness of the body movements and skeletal schema, as well as to access and explore sensorial information.

A major source of inspiration on this theme was the work of Émile Coué, who, in the first decade of the twentieth century, introduced a method of psychotherapy using positive and optimistic autosuggestion as a form of therapy for self-healing and self-improvement.[i] Feldenkrais was very impressed by Coué's work, and in 1929 he translated into Hebrew a book introducing the method that describes how hundreds of people visited Coué's clinic, and how through autosuggestion many were relieved of their ailments.[ii]

---

[i] For the stimulating effect that the work of Émile Coué de la Châtaigneraie had on Feldenkrais, see Reese 2015, chap. 2.

[ii] *The Practice of Autosuggestion by the Method of Émile Coué*. Originally published in English by C. Harry Brooks. The foreword to the Hebrew translation was written by the Israeli philosopher Shmuel Hugo Bergman.

The power of autosuggestion to positively affect body health attracted Feldenkrais's attention, but it was rather the power of self-improvement that was his main interest. He added two chapters to the book as an epilogue, and in the opening words to the chapter "The Unconscious as Executor," he makes clear that he will not be dealing with how to alleviate pain or ease the heavy burden that sick people carry.[i] Feldenkrais's intention is different. He writes:

> Using examples from real life, we will demonstrate that using autosuggestion we can achieve far superior results rather than merely being in a condition no worse than someone else.[ii]

In Coué's method, Feldenkrais identified an activity or faculty that can reach deep into the organism and has the power to change its course. Feldenkrais saw in autosuggestion a power that enables access to nonconscious processes, to the organism's archives, and facilitates improvement and self-change. To achieve a higher goal than not being "worse than someone else" is both an inspiration and a purpose at the heart of the Feldenkrais Method, as a call for constant growth and expansion.

---

[i] The two chapters that Feldenkrais added to his translation were later translated into English, and published as the monograph *Thinking and Doing*. The titles are "The Unconscious as Executor" and "Last in Deed, First in Thought." The Hebrew term used by Feldenkrais for "unconscious" is בלתי-הכרתי, which literally means "not-knowable." He does not use תת-מודע or בלתי-מודע, which stand for subconscious and unconscious, respectively. The meaning of the term he uses is analogous to the term "nonconscious" used in the neuroscientific context. See note ii on p. 45.

[ii] *Thinking and Doing*. p.1.

For a lasting improvement, the Feldenkrais Method considers it necessary to elicit information from the sensorial nonconscious. Indeed, the method is built on the axiom that nonconscious processes carry a reservoir of information that can be accessed through somatic practices. The reservoir contains the memories of the history of the body and the skeletal schema, from the primitive reflexes to the generation of habitual movements—a record of how the process of learning to move developed throughout the years.

Coué considered imagination, rather than the will, as an all-embracing connection between the mind and the body, and as a channel to access body processes. Feldenkrais adopted Coué's view that "Our actions spring not from our Will, but from our Imagination." Indeed, in many lessons, especially the mainly meditative ones, there is autosuggestive modus blended with the imagination that has a hypnotic effect of sorts, with the aim of accessing those memories. Scanning the body, focusing the attention on the self-image, is done guided by the slow and soothing voice of the practitioner, inviting the participants to watch for regular breathing, to relax, and to leave aside all effort and tension of the muscles. Imagination serves to amplify the internal sensing of the body and to support the meditative scanning that refines the self-image.

The weight that imagination has in the Feldenkrais Method cannot be overstated. This is succinctly expressed in the following words:

> In this lesson you will learn to use a group of muscles for a specific movement in various positions of the body. You will make the joints employed in this movement more flexible and reach the anatomically possible limits within the first hour. You will learn the effect of movements of the head on muscular tension, the effect of imagined movement on real movement,

and to inhibit verbalization in imagined movement—all of which leads to completion of the body image. You will also be able to transfer improvement actively obtained by one side of the body to the other inactive side, which did not take part in the movement, by means of visualization or thought only.[i]

What is noticeable in this paragraph is that Feldenkrais considers the blend of thought with visualization, which equals imagination, a means to expand and spread the freedom, organization, and integration achieved in one part of the body to another—making imagination one of the engines of self-change, and supplementing how change and transformation can be attained (chapter 9).

At a first glance, granting imagination such power might be surprising; however, today we have sufficient evidence from cutting-edge research in neuroscience that intending or imagining body movements recreates actual movements. It has been shown that thinking of, and even watching, movement produces similar brain activity to performing it.

The pioneers of these findings were the Italian investigators Vittorio Gallese and Giacomo Rizzolatti, who in a series of remarkable papers report their discovery of "mirror neurons" in the premotor cortex of monkeys. Using microelectrodes that recorded from individual neurons, they observed that the same neuron "fired" (i.e., emitted an action potential, or nerve impulse) both when the monkey grasped an object, such as a raisin, and when the monkey witnessed another monkey performing the same action. Self-initiated actions and watching another individual perform the identical action evoke the same

---

[i] *Awareness Through Movement*, p. 130.

neural response. Mirror neurons fire, not in all actions, but rather in response to the performance of intentional acts.[i] Later research has shown that the brain also predicts what feeling will follow if the imagined movements are executed.[ii] Feldenkrais could envisage that imagining movements activates all the neuromotor aspects of the movements themselves.

Imagining – The Lessons

The Feldenkrais Method uses imagination to enhance somatic awareness in two main ways. One is when the instructions are to imagine doing a sequence of movements before actually doing them, or instead of doing them. The other way is when imagination is a central theme of the lesson. In the former, the imaginary movements are done with any part of the body, such as shoulder, hip, or leg, or with one side of the body. In the latter case, imagination usually comes in support of meditative scanning and to refine the self-image.

Some of the lessons of the former kind are "Minimal Movements; Lying on the Side, Begin the Movements in Imagination,"[iii] and "Imagination and Action to Complete the Back–Self Image,"[iv] in which the initial movements are made in the imagination. In "Length and Fists" imagination is used to sense the arms as being of equal length, and the fists as of equal size, even though they felt like they were different sizes

---

[i] Gallese et al. 1996, Rizzolatti and Arbib 1998, Rizzolatti 2005.

[ii] Kilteni et al. 2018.

[iii] AY 232 – (Reel 16/4/3).

[iv] E 46. This lesson is not included in Stransky's transcripts.

due to the specific configuration of the body during the lesson.[i] In lessons "Foot on the Head,"[ii] and "Classic Rotation Sitting,"[iii] the movements of one side of the body are done in the imagination, and in "Foot on the Head" Feldenkrais refers to the imaginary part of the lesson as "the most important part of this lesson."[iv]

We have seen above how the imaginational elements are staged in some of the lessons; worth mentioning is "Scanning,"[v] where two imaginary fingers press along the spine, and an imaginary iron ball rolls through all parts of the back of the body in great detail. In lessons "A Lecture/Lesson: Self-image Lecture, the Line of a Ball that Rolls,"[vi] "Imagination and Action to Complete the Back–Self Image,"[vii] and "Becoming Aware of Parts of Which We are not Conscious with the Help of Those of Which We are Conscious,"[viii] the imaginary motifs are the engine of the movements and of the sensorial layer, whether it is an imaginary finger pressing the spine vertebra by vertebra; a ball traveling throughout the back, along its different parts, and in diagonal lines; or an imaginary lifting of the foot and hand. In "Knots," it is an imaginary rope tied around different parts of the body, with the

---

[i] AY 347 – (Reel 23/4/2).

[ii] AY 034 – (Reel 3/3/1).

[iii] Lesson 3, in *San Francisco Evening Class Notes*.

[iv] For more and different uses of imagination in the lessons, search the word "imagine" in Feldy Notebook, https://feldynotebook.com.

[v] E 2/Es 1.

[vi] AY 303 – (Reel 21/1/3).

[vii] E 46.

[viii] ATM Lesson 11.

knot of the rope moving around, that stimulates those parts,[i] and in "Primary Image,"[ii] imagination is used to represent the body-image as a geometrical construct.

In the series of lessons "The Line of Effort in the Back in Lifting,"[iii] "The Line of Effort in the Stomach and the Chest,"[iv] and "The Line of Effort in Lying on the Back,"[v] there is little movement, while an imaginary hand touches parts of the body, applying pressure to feel the bones. In these lessons an imaginary heavy iron ball exerts pressure while slowly rolling throughout the back or front of the body, demarcating a "line of effort" that reveals the optimal path of force through the skeleton. Imagination is also a tool to mark the lateralization of the body into right and left, by means of an imaginary plane passing through the body at the midline, in "A Plane Dividing the Body #1,"[vi] and "A Plane Dividing the Body #2."[vii]

In sum, imagination has the power to prompt brain connections and sensorial access to parts of the body and movements that are concealed, nonconscious, or not active. Imagination expands and deepens the range of sensory awareness

---

[i] AY 337 – (Reel 23/1/5).

[ii] AY 338 – (Reel 23/2/1).

[iii] AY 305 – (Reel 21/2/1).

[iv] AY 306 – (Reel 21/2/2).

[v] AY 307 – (Reel 21/2/3).

[vi] AY 212 – (Reel 9/1/3).

[vii] AY 115 – (Reel 9/1/6).

PART FOUR

THE SCIENCE OF SELF-TRANSFORMATION

Overture

In its early years, when it was in the process of gestation and diffusion, the Feldenkrais Method attracted the attention of students, researchers, and scientists from different spheres of knowledge, as well as people from the arts.[i] Interest has been growing ever since, and during the last decades we have witnessed a significant expansion of the number of participants, as well as of the fields of knowledge finding value in the method.[ii] The method has an unparalleled magnetic force, attracting the attention of participants and researchers from the humanities and the arts, as well as from the social and exact sciences.

Nowadays the Feldenkrais Method is included in the curricula of prestigious theatre and dance academies, and doctoral theses and books are being written on the method's intersection with the arts.[iii] Similarly, scientists of diverse disciplines have recognized the wisdom of the Feldenkrais Method, at a time when technological and methodological innovations have made it possible to corroborate, with evidence-based research, some of the method's beneficial effects on movement, health, and behavior.[iv]

---

[i] For Feldenkrais and theatre, see Reese 2015, chap. 6.

[ii] The IFF Research Group is a group of Feldenkrais practitioners with diverse research backgrounds that promotes scientific knowledge in relation to the Feldenkrais Method, https://sites.google.com/feldenkrais-method.org/researchgroup.

[iii] See Hancock 2015, Fredricksson 2017, Ciofu 2018, Sholl 2021.

[iv] In Google Scholar, a search for "Feldenkrais Therapy" finds more than 8,000 articles published in peer-reviewed scientific journals and in books. Accessed May 11, 2022.

It is reasonable to believe that further research will expand our knowledge about the method's applications and its benefits, which encompass a wide range of human experience, from physical and mental health to creative fields such as the performing arts. The challenge of providing a scientific basis for the method, however, is not simple, given that in the Feldenkrais Method there is a confluence of diverse spheres of knowledge, including physiology, anatomy, physics, neuroscience, body mechanics, kinesiology, and somatic studies. The Feldenkrais Method branches into somatic psychology and body therapeutics as well.

With this book, I wish to contribute to such effort with an analysis of the scientific basis, and its application in the process of self-change, inherent in the Feldenkrais Method. The analysis is informed by the principles of sensorimotor development, the role that primitive reflexes play in such a process, as well as the dynamics of habit formation in behavior and in the brain. I have added, as well, scientific research evidencing the dynamics at work in the process of transformation. One instance is research on chronic pain and on the phantom limb, which supports the theme of organismic or material-sensorial memory that orchestrates the body movements (chapter 3). In another instance, I refer to the research on mirror neurons, which shows that imagination and intention trigger the same nervous and brain processes that actual movements activate (chapter 11)—attesting to imagination's power to actively participate in the process of transformation.

A field that doubtlessly will deepen and broaden the scientific mantle of the Feldenkrais Method is neuroscience.[i] In the following I will be looking at two lines of thought where neuroscience meets the

---

[i] See Doidge 2015.

Feldenkrais Method. The first theme is the interaction between consciousness and nonconscious processes; the second is neuroplasticity. These are two areas that intersect with the Feldenkrais Method, and in addition to giving us a glance at the method from the perspective of the brain, they position the Feldenkrais Method on the frontiers of science, particularly in kinesiology and somatosensory studies.[i]

Sensorial Consciousness

We described the changes that the Feldenkrais Method generates as a process of revisiting and resetting the skeletal schema and movement patterns that have become automatized, not fully integrated during early motor development, or dysfunctional in later life. These patterns affect the gait, range of movement, flexibility, and suppleness of the body, and become integral to the self-image, to its quality. The line of argument has been, essentially, that the Feldenkrais Method is a somatic practice that stimulates the roots of motor development and the ensuing organization of the body, its posture(s) and its movements, as well as restructuring habitual movement patterns. While doing this, it puts forward alternative movements for the same action, thereby reattuning the sensorimotor layer, and with it, the self-image. With this process, the functionality of the body's movements is partially or fully restored.

This thesis raises an essential question: How is the retrieving possible? How does a somatic practice repossess unconscious information and memories? How should we understand the correlation between

---

[i] A Google Scholar search on "Feldenkrais" and "Neuroscience" finds more than 2,000 entries. Accessed Oct. 10, 2021.

consciousness or awareness and nonconscious processes? While Feld-enkrais asserts "that sensory stimuli are closer to our unconscious, sub-conscious, or autonomous functioning than any of our conscious un-derstanding,"[i] he still does not tell us more about it.

These questions fall within the realm of neuroscience and brain studies in general. To face them, I will consider some major tenets of the work of Antonio Damasio. Damasio's work is extensive, encom-passing a whole panoply of neurobiology and theoretical work. I will not refer here to his vast experimental research, but rather to the conclu-sions of a central piece of his work concerning the dynamics between consciousness and nonconsciousness.

In his investigation of the bio-mechanism that constructs con-sciousness, Damasio follows an evolutionary path that includes the development of the brain both in the human species and in the indi-vidual. His aim is to reveal the process from which consciousness arises in human beings—or, for that matter, in any organism—and how it evolves in every individual.

Damasio finds a leading role of unconscious or nonconscious processes in their interaction with consciousness and action.[ii] The nonconscious is vital for the very existence of the organism, given how much of the information that any life-form has to process to reg-ulate the basic functions of life and to preserve itself is nonconscious. Moreover, nonconscious processes have the essential function of providing a foundation for the activities of consciousness, or, in other words, of being the fertile ground where knowledge grows. Indeed,

---

[i] *The Elusive Obvious*, p. 3.

[ii] For nonconscious, unconscious, and subconscious, see note ii on page 45

for Damasio, the knowledge base of human beings is *"implicit, encrypted,* and *unconscious"* (emphasis in original).[i]

Damasio's intention is not to downgrade consciousness, but rather to upgrade nonconsciousness. Indeed, he regards nonconsciousness as holding an enormous reservoir of information and knowledge, as well as archiving our memories. These include "memory of things, of properties of things, of persons... of biological regulations"; "all of our memory, inherited from evolution and available at birth or acquired through learning thereafter."[ii] Indeed, nonconscious memories harbor "our own past, and often the past of our biological species and of culture."[iii]

Written eighty years earlier, Feldenkrais's words on the unconscious are almost identical. Like Damasio, he upgrades the nonconscious without downgrading consciousness, and regards the nonconscious as "a veritable storehouse of memories and knowledge that can become available to us only through diligent observation, study, experience, and much effort."[iv] And, like Damasio, he regards the nonconscious as "the repository not only of our own personal memories and experiences, but also of those of our fathers and forefathers over many generations of experience and repetition."[v]

Given the great similarity, it is not surprising that the conclusions reached by Damasio's research are fully compatible with the main principles on which the power of self-transformation of the Feldenkrais Method rests. Indeed, Damasio's findings on the dynamics

---

[i] Damasio 2010, p. 144.

[ii] Damasio 1999, p. 332.

[iii] Damasio 2010, p. 133.

[iv] *Thinking and Doing,* p. 35.

[v] Ibid., p. 34.

between consciousness and nonconsciousness support the modus operandi of the Feldenkrais Method in its pursuit of self-transformation. We can best appreciate this consonance in relation to the primitive reflexes and the habits.[i]

Neonatal and primitive reflexes are, certainly, part of the nonconscious information that the organism owns for the management of life, self-preservation, and self-protection. It is information carried by the human organism from the evolutionary process and encrypted in the nervous system of every person. These reflexes are the fertile ground for knowing how to move, how to roll, to sit up, to crawl, to stand up, and to walk, by their conversion from involuntary to voluntary movements over the course of development. They are, as well, the ground for the other layers that grow from the sensorial: feelings and thoughts (chapter 6).

In Damasio's research and theory, the nonconscious is a dynamic repository where information can be stored as well as retrieved. This description corresponds to the Feldenkrais Method's conception of habits as raw material for the process of self-transformation (chapter 7).

Damasio explains that many conscious processes are, at some point in time, transferred from the "conscious space" to another

---

[i] To be sure, Feldenkrais uses the term "awareness" while Damasio uses the term "consciousness"; both, however, have very similar meanings. For Feldenkrais "awareness" is used to denote "consciousness-of plus knowledge" (*Awareness Through Movement*, p. 95), which stands for somatic consciousness, a sensorial knowledge of the body by the body, as "my movements," "my posture," "my feelings," "my thoughts," and "my self-image." For Damasio "consciousness is a state of mind in which there is knowledge of one's own existence and of the existence of surroundings" (Damasio 2010, p.157). Both of them coincide in regarding their concepts as dispositions with both a knowledge and a self-knowledge component.

network of the brain that harbors the nonconscious, where they continue to be major components of our behavior and the decisions we make. This is a nonconscious autopilot of sorts that allows us "to walk home without consciously focusing on the route."[i] Another example of habitual practices that Damasio gives is that of learned skills, which he describes in the following way:

> Outsourcing expertise to the nonconscious space is what we do when we hone a skill so finely that we are no longer aware of the technical steps needed to be skillful. We develop skills in the clear light of consciousness, but then we let them go underground, into the roomy basement of our minds, where they do not clutter the exiguous square footage of conscious reflection space.[ii]

This is, indeed, what happens when a practice becomes habitual, whether it is walking after converting the primitive reflexes into voluntary movements or playing a musical instrument. After we master the movements, we can perform them without thinking about the initial steps of how we learned them. That information, however, is not erased. In the case of sensorimotor development, it has been genetically inherited from our ancestors, and is waiting to be transmitted to our descendants. The information goes "to the roomy basement of our minds," which is none other than the nonconscious.

The store of memory that we keep in the nonconscious, Damasio adds, "exists in dispositional form (a synonym for *implicit, covert,*

---

[i] Damasio 2010, p. 164.

[ii] Ibid., p. 275.

nonconscious), waiting to become an explicit image or action [emphasis in original]."[i] "Images," here, refers to representations in our mind of events located outside of the brain, and the term refers not just to the visual kind, but to "images of any sense origin such as auditory, visceral, tactile, and so forth."[ii] Although Damasio does not tell us what specific practices or doings convert implicit to explicit images, he does tell us such practices' general function: "making the images *ours*" [emphasis in original].[iii]

Bringing this nonconscious information, these memories and recollections, back from Damasio's "roomy basement of the mind" or from Feldenkrais's "storehouse" to their rightful owner—the singular, bounded organism—is at the heart of the process of self-transformation of the Feldenkrais Method. We can thus see how the Feldenkrais Method is one of those practices or actions of retrieval and revivification that Damasio's theory delineates, as a practice of kinesthetic-somatic awareness and self-appropriation, when images of our movements, and the actions themselves, become genuine parts of ourselves.

Brain Plasticity

The central idea of this book is that the Feldenkrais Method shows us how to functionally integrate our body movements and sensorial layers, as an active force of self-making, self-sustaining, and self-transformation. The changes can be temporary, but with regular and

---

[i] Damasio 1999, p. 332.

[ii] Damasio 2010, p.18.

[iii] Ibid., p. 10.

sufficient practice, and a concurrent process of somatic awareness, they become lasting functional modifications that rewire the movements in the brain and nervous system and transform the self-image.

That changes in the body, in the way we move, and in the practices we engage in modify our brain wiring is little wonder. This is something that we all experience during life transitions from childhood to adolescence and adulthood. We also experience such changes on a variety of occasions when we engage in new activities, whether mental, emotional, or physical: learning a new language, acquiring new skills, falling in love, parenting, emigrating to another country, or adapting to a new situation.

Brain plasticity, or *neuroplasticity*, is the ability of the brain to change its own set of connections and its functioning throughout an individual's life. The brain's capacity to change is a fact researched and evidenced by neuroscience since the second half of the twentieth century.[i] Researchers then found that the brain's ability to change is not limited to the modifications that accompany and adapt to the new conditions a "regular" course of life presents and requires, such as puberty or parenthood. Plasticity also applies to functions of the brain that are impaired or completely lost either in an accident, through illness, or by suffering a traumatic experience. The paradigm-changing finding was that brain activity associated with a given function can be transferred to a different location in the brain. Consequently, brain injury doesn't necessarily eliminate the possibility of activating the part of the body linked to the site of the injury, and functionality of body movements or faculties can often be fully or partially restored.

---

[i] The first to use and define the term "neuroplasticity" was the Polish neuroscientist Jerzy Konorsky, in 1948.

Before the plasticity of the brain was scientifically established by theory and research, the conventional view and scientific paradigm had two major tenets: first, that brain activity is localized, linked to brain areas genetically hardwired to perform specific functions, and to those alone. That is, when we speak, it is the speech area of the brain that is active; when we recall something, it is the memory area that is active; and when we see, it is the visual area that is active. Once one of the areas is damaged, it cannot be replaced, and the function is partially or fully lost. The second principle was that the brain reached physical and functional maturity largely in the first year of life. After that, the maturation of brain cells and the "wiring" of the brain were thought to be fixed.

Research has shown that both tenets are inaccurate. First, the entire cortex, not just the area responsible for a certain function, is activated when a given task is initiated. Indeed, neuroplasticity can be observed at multiple scales, from microscopic changes in individual neurons to larger-scale changes such as cortical remapping in response to injury. Second, even though the developing brain exhibits a higher degree of plasticity than the adult brain, many aspects of the brain can be altered throughout adulthood.

At the time when Feldenkrais conceptualized his method, neuroscience did not have the support of the groundbreaking technologies it has today, such as positron emission tomography (PET) scanning and functional magnetic resonance imaging (fMRI), which have exponentially advanced our knowledge of the brain.[i] The non-plasticity

---

[i] For example, lesions in the brain caused by neurological disease, a topic central in brain research, used to be revealed only at the time of autopsy, often many years after the study was initiated. Today, thanks to technical

(localist) theory was then the established paradigm. Nevertheless, Feldenkrais built his method having the idea of neuroplasticity in mind before it had a name or a proposed mechanism: on various occasions he expressed his full disagreement with the idea that the brain is a static organ that doesn't change after the so-called maturation period.[i]

Already during the years when the Feldenkrais Method was starting to spread in the United States, the neuroscientist Karl Pribram had a prescient insight into the method's effects on the brain, from observing the changes it made in body movements and in human functioning in general. Pribram recognized the innovative brain-changing importance of the method. He could envisage the effectiveness of the method in changing brain maps and connections, and is commonly quoted as saying that "Feldenkrais is not just pushing muscles around, but changing things in the brain itself."[ii]

The changes in neurological mapping that the Feldenkrais Method generates are still uncharted territory, and evidence of this sort is not coming soon. Even so, research is being done in different venues, and several practitioners have incorporated the theme of neuroplasticity into their practice and teachings. Worth mentioning is David Zemach-Bersin, who has effectively integrated the neuroplasticity innovations into his Functional Integration classes and seminars, and Anat Baniel,

---

developments, lesions can be analyzed in a 3D reconstruction of the living patient's brain.

[i] See Feldenkrais's introduction to *Body and Mature Behavior*, and AM 1 – Week 2 – June 20 AM 1: "Talk: Crawling and Brain Functions."

[ii] For more on this theme, listen to "The Feldenkrais–Pribram Discussions."

who blends brain-plasticity hindsight with the main guidelines of the Feldenkrais Method.[i]

One of the world's leading neuroscientists who have expressed an opinion on the method is Michael Merzenich. In his research, Merzenich has shown in rich scientific detail how our brain's processing areas change under certain conditions, practices, and interactions. He and his teams of researchers have used their neuroplastic innovations to improve many people's abilities to think and perceive, by redesigning specific brain maps.[ii]

In a short interview in which he referred to the Feldenkrais Method, Merzenich deems it fully compatible with his views, and considers his own "evolution on thinking about brain plasticity as very consistent with the Feldenkrais Method."[iii] Indeed, Merzenich views the practice of the Feldenkrais Method as being in full agreement with his theory of brain plasticity and with current neuroscience in general.

Merzenich draws an interesting parallel and complementarity between the Feldenkrais Method and neuroscience. He praises the ability of Feldenkrais Method practitioners who "by looking at the movement of a person can see the distortions, the inadequacy of the movements." Neuroscience, he affirms, "understands and knows where those distortions or deficiencies come from, and the Feldenkrais Method has the ability to understand how to deal with them."

---

[i] Baniel 2012. For improvements in cognitive and attentional skills through mindful practice of movements, see Clark et al. 2015.

[ii] Michael Merzenich is a professor emeritus neuroscientist at the University of California, San Francisco, and creator of BrainHQ online brain-learning software.

[iii] See https://www.youtube.com/watch?v=rupZ-wlRdA0.

Merzenich identifies one of the main messages of the Feldenkrais Method when he comments that in practicing the Feldenkrais Method, "quite rapidly the person understands that they have the capacity to change." This, he adds, is in full accord with what brain retraining studies show: "When we talk about motivation and change, we are talking about neurology."[i] Merzenich thus puts the Feldenkrais Method and neuroscience on a complementary footing in regard to self-change.

One of the themes that Merzenich appreciates is the compatibility he sees between the Feldenkrais Method and the optimal conditions for the brain's functioning. When making any movement, even just moving from one place or position to another, having more available alternatives, more different ways to do the action, "is what the brain wants." The Feldenkrais Method responds to the needs of the brain by looking for alternative pathways for an action that lead to a change, an improvement, and increased flexibility in responding to a changing world. In the process, one does nothing less than draw, redraw, and renovate brain maps.

Merzenich's book, *Soft-Wired*, carries another important message. The possibility of changing how the brain is wired is, for him, tied to the idea of enriching the quality of life at any age. He writes that people have "a remarkable built-in ability to strengthen and grow the person that you are, at any age."[ii] The self-change process that aspires to a true(r) self is open to anyone at any stage of life.

---

[i] Ibid.

[ii] Merzenich 2013, p.20.

Concern for Oneself and for Others

The Feldenkrais Method is not usually linked to a moral or ethical commitment; nevertheless, it has one. I have proposed elsewhere to use the concept "care of the self," as developed by the philosopher Michel Foucault, to shed light on the ethical aspects of the method.[i] Foucault borrowed the concept from the ancient Greek philosophers, and explained that while the ancient motto "Know thyself" has been adopted in modern times, we have forgotten that for the Greeks this also implied "care of the self."[ii]

Care of the self is a sensibility through which individuals value being conscious of their own thoughts and attitudes, and participate in practices aimed at raising awareness of the highest state of the self. These practices are meant to be focused on oneself, and doing so, says Foucault, is the means to "take responsibility for oneself and by which one changes, transforms, and even transfigures oneself."[iii] The process of self-change of the Feldenkrais Method carries such a message—a call to take responsibility for oneself so as to heal, or better, transform oneself in a way that is truthful to the embodied self.

The care of the self also carries a responsibility toward others: Foucault describes it as an attitude "towards the self, others, and the world."[iv] This is a message that the Feldenkrais Method carries as well. In the same measure that Feldenkrais was troubled by the consequences that

---

[i] Mansbach 2015.

[ii] Foucault 1988a.

[iii] Foucault 2005, p. 11-12.

[iv] Ibid., p. 10.

stagnation at a personal level can have for any individual, he was also concerned about stagnation in the social sphere. He considered "the immutability of the social laws, habits, and traditions themselves"[i] the cause that had brought the society in which he lived, and the social structure and economic conditions that sustained it, to a conservatism that hindered the achievement of a better life and a better society. On this theme he wrote:

> While expecting hopefully that the environment will be changed by our collective efforts, we must also make sure that everything amenable to human influence in each individual is used to facilitate adaptation. This will not only eliminate much misery in the present generation but will also give a better chance to the next.[ii]

It would be fair to say that Feldenkrais saw the flexibility acquired through his method, and the self-changing dynamics of his lessons, as a way to facilitate the adaptation to the pulse of life that he deemed necessary for a better life. He regarded the possibility of change inherent in every person, sustained by the change of habits and of the most deep-rooted behavior, as a moving gear in the dynamics of change in society that carries a responsibility for others and for future generations.

It is interesting to notice that the two-tiered responsibility that the process of self-change carries, as a responsibility for oneself and for others, also has an evolutional-neurological correlate, where consciousness, rather than care, is at the center. On this theme Damasio writes:

---

[i] *Body and Mature Behavior*, p. 10.
[ii] Ibid., p. 11.

At its simplest and most basic level, consciousness lets us recognize an irresistible urge to stay alive and develop a concern for the self. At its most complex and elaborate level, consciousness helps us develop concern for other selves and improve the art of life.[i]

Through the prisms of both ethics and neuroscience, we can see the Feldenkrais Method as an art of self-fashioning in which agency blends with responsibility for oneself and others, enacting needs and drives of the organism and the brain itself while promoting the growth and integration of the embodied self.

---

[i] Damasio 1999, p. 5.

Acknowledgments

More than two decades ago, I discovered the Feldenkrais Method through my work in philosophy, though not in the way you might think. I had been writing a book on one of the most intricate German philosophers, sitting at my desk for long hours every day over almost four years, expecting to receive my university tenure with its publication. At the end of writing that book, a disc in my neck became herniated, and a nerve lesioned. I tried all the painkillers available over the counter and by prescription, including strong opiates, yet with no results. The medical specialists I consulted suggested that the only solution would be surgery, which I refused. So I set out to seek alternative cures, and that is how the Feldenkrais Method came into play for me.

Daphna Alexandrovich, a Feldenkrais practitioner in Jerusalem, gave me a series of Functional Integration lessons that helped to ease the pain, enabled me to walk and lie down again, and restored mobility to the affected arm and my neck. I continued practicing with Daphna for some time, during which she encouraged me to enroll in a Feldenkrais Method training course—and I did. For all this, I am infinitely grateful to her.

In the course of my training in Israel and advanced workshops abroad, I had the opportunity to meet a variety of wonderful and stimulating teachers. I wish to thank them all, in particular, Beatriz Walterspiel, Anat Krivine, and Eilat Almagor, who, each with her expertise and distinct didactic style and tone, taught me the nuances and the potential reaches of the method. In retrospect, I realize that I learned just as much from the other trainees and participants by observing their body dynamics, noticing the different skeletal configurations, and practicing FI technique with them. I thank each of my co-learners for sharing such enriching body experiences, which became a major source of inspiration for this book.

I consider myself lucky to have found in Annie Gottlieb a particularly skillful editor who is also a highly perceptive Feldenkrais Professional Training Program graduate. I wish to thank her for making this book eminently more readable than it might have been otherwise and much more accurate in describing the lessons.

I am extremely grateful to my dear friend Susanne Kunjappu-Jellinek, an amazing visual artist and the greatest cover designer I could ever imagine.

My deepest thanks to David Zemach-Bersin for his enthusiastic encouragement, valuable advice, and constructive comments on this book.

Many thanks to the archive of the International Feldenkrais Federation (IFF) for allowing me the opportunity to browse through the manuscripts of Moshe Feldenkrais's books and lectures. Special thanks to Kai Schaper for his kindness and help, and Allegra Heidelinde for her diligent assembling of a collection of lessons accompanying this book.

Finally, I want to thank my life partner, Carola, for being a passionate companion and friend during this exciting journey. Without her support and trust, I cannot imagine having written this book. Immeasurable gratitude and love go to her.

About the Author

Abraham Mansbach is a philosopher and a Feldenkrais practitioner. Born in Mexico City in 1949, he has lived in Israel since 1976. After his undergraduate studies in economics at the Instituto Tecnológico Autónomo de México (ITAM), he completed his graduate studies in philosophy at the Hebrew University of Jerusalem (M.A. and Ph.D.) and The New School for Social Research, New York (postdoctoral research). He received his certification as a Feldenkrais practitioner from the Israeli Feldenkrais Association.

Professionally, Abraham is a professor emeritus of philosophy at the Ben-Gurion University of the Negev (Israel), and has been practicing the Feldenkrais Method for more than two decades, including teaching and directing workshops at venues in Europe (Spain and Germany) and Mexico. In his private practice in Israel he works with groups and in person-to-person lessons with people interested in self-healing and transformation.

In his philosophical work, Abraham specializes in the relationship between identity, selfhood, and the body, and, more specifically, in the ways in which practices shape persons and their identities. His books and scholarly articles are phenomenological studies of basic human experiences, such as being in the world and using tools, as well as of artistic creation and practices that are exercised in the public sphere, such as truth-telling (whistleblowing). Most recently, he has published on intersections of the Feldenkrais Method with the cultural domain as representative of a wider "somatic turn" of Western culture.

Abraham's work has been published widely in academic journals, and his publications are quoted extensively in books and professional journals of diverse fields of knowledge. In Israel, his work has been highly praised, and he has received grants for his research from a variety of sources, among them the Richard Koebner Minerva Center, the Edmond Rothschild Foundation, and The Israel Science Foundation (ISF), founded by the Israel Academy of Sciences and Humanities.

Index of Awareness Through Movement (ATM) Lessons

Amherst Training Course (Recordings)

AM 1 – Week 1 – June 9 AM1: Sucking – Life's First Movement 70

AM 1 – Week 2 – June 16 AM2: Rolling With Entire Self.........................56

AM 1 – Week 2 – June 17 AM1: Seated and Twist Left (part 1)
["Dead Bird"].. 75

AM 1 – Week 2 – June 20 AM1: Talk: Crawling and Brain Functions.....58, 135

AM 1 – Week 3 – June 23 AM1: Lying on Stomach (continued).................. 7

AM 1 – Week 7 – July 24 AM1: Morning Prayer...............................112

AM 2 – Week 1 – June 10 PM2: On Back Flexing Torso/Bell Crawl..............82

AM 2 – Week 1 – June 11 AM1: Swimming Crawl/Bell Hand, Think Toes...82

AM 2 – Week 1 – June 11 AM2: Swimming Crawl/Bell Hand, Think
    Toes (cont'd.)..82

Alexander Yanai Collections

AY 003: Rolling to Sit With the Elbows – (Reel 1/2/2)...........................54

AY 017: Breathing – (Reel 2/2/2)............................. 109

AY 021: Contracting the Abdomen While Exhaling – (Reel 2/3/2)............109

AY 023: Palate, Mouth, and Teeth – (Reel 2/3/5)..............................108

AY 024 The Body Image, a Lecture – (Reels 2/4/1 and 2/4/3)................3, 25

AY 041: Basic Bending – (Reel 3/4/4)...75

AY 046: Lowering the Head – (Reel 4/1/4) 111

AY 050: Lowering the Head – (Reel 4/2/4)....................................111

AY 057: Lifting the Head on All Fours – (Reel 4/4/2)........................61, 80

AY 058: Transferring Support While on the Stomach – (Reel 4/4/3)........77

AY 067: Lengthening the Leg Into Pulling Movements While
Rolling – (Reel 5/4/1)..55, 95

AY 068: Rolling the Fists – (Reel 5/4/2)......................................71

AY 076: Slow Lifting; on the Stomach – (Reel 6/2/5)........................ .77

AY 078: Standing – (Reel 6/3/2)..88

AY 099: Lifting the Elbows With a Loose Hand – (Reel 8/1/3....................58

AY 112: A Plane Dividing the Body #1 – (Reel 9/1/3) 74, 121

AY 115: A Plane Dividing the Body #2 – (Reel 9/1/6) 74, 121

AY 122: Rolling Right and Left – (Reel 9/3/1) 50

AY 123: On the Knees; Diagonal See-Saw – (Reel 9/3/6).........................62

AY 138: Walking on the Heels – (Reel 10/2/4)..92

AY 145: From Sitting to Standing While Turning – (Reel 10/4/3)..............96

AY 165: The Eyeball Lesson – (Reel 12/2/1) 108

AY 172: Stopping the Breath – (Reel 12/3/5).................................. 109

AY 177: Making the Spine Flexible and Integrating It – (Reel 13/1/1)......80

AY 178: Lengthening the Arms – (Reel 13/1/2)..52

AY 222: On the Abdomen, a Hand Lifting the Head – (Reel 16/1/1).….......78

AY 223: Rolling From the Back to Side-Sitting – (Reel 16/1/2)......... 54

AY 234: Standing Backward, #1 – (Reel 17/1/1).......................................64

AY 235: Standing (Shaking in the Heels) – (Reel 17/1/2)..........................64

AY 238: Standing Backward, #2 – (Reel 17/2/1) 64

AY 274: Introduction to Walking 1 – (Reel 19/2/4) 65

AY 275: Introduction to Walking 2 continuation – (Reel 19/2/5)..............65

AY 283: Continuation on One Leg – (Reel 19/4/3) 88

AY 289: Standing on One Leg With Movements – (Reel 20/2/1) 89

AY 303: A Lecture/Lesson: Self-image Lecture, the Line of a Ball that Rolls –
(Reel 21/1/3) 15, 23, 26, 120

AY 305: The Line of Effort in the Back in Lifting – (Reel 21/2/1)..............121

AY 306: The Line of Effort in the Stomach and the Chest – (Reel 21/2/2)....121

AY 307: The Line of Effort in Lying on the Back – (Reel 21/2/3)...............121

AY 313: Rolling at the Rate of Stretching and Bending –
(Reel 21/4/1)..50, 82

AY 322: In Sitting, Lengthening the Arms – (Reel 22/2/2) 73

AY 326: Sitting – Lying – (Reel 22/3/2) 94

AY 327: Sitting – Lying, continuation – (Reel 22/3/3).........................53, 94

AY 337: Knots (Reel 23/1/5) 20, 121

AY 338: Primary Image – (Reel 23/2/1)..21, 121
AY 339: Simpler – (Reel 23/2/2) 22, 107
AY 345: Diagonal Image – (Reel 23/3/4) 74
AY 354: Walking Backward – (Reel 24/2/1) 97
AY 363: Prayer – (Reel 24/3/2) 112
AY 370: Lifting the Head – (Reel 24/3/9) 80
AY 417: Preparation for Rolling to Sitting – (Reel 27/2/1) 55, 95
AY 420: In Sitting – Twisting With the Eyes – (Reel 27/2/4).....................75
AY 484: In Standing, Turning With the Eyes – (Reel 31/3/3).....................89
AY 496: The Face – (Reel 32/3/2) 107
AY 501: Introduction to Walking – (Reel 33/1/1) 67, 90
AY 502: Walking and Crawling – (Reel 33/1/2) 66, 90
AY 503: Hoping and Arms – (Reel 33/1/3) 91
AY 504: Continuation and Return – (Reel 33/1/4) 92
AY 512: Fish Swimming – (Reel 33/3/3)..59
AY 513: Reptiles – (Reel 33/3/4) 60
AY 515: Dragging Knees to the Stomach – (Reel 33/4/1) 59
AY 528: Advancing on All Fours – (Reel 34/3/2) 63

Awareness Through Movement: Easy-to-Do Health Exercises to Improve Your Posture, Vision, Imagination, and Personal Awareness. (Book)

Lesson 4: Differentiation of Parts and Functions in Breathing..................110
Lesson 11: Becoming Aware of Parts of Which We are not Conscious With the
    Help of Those of Which We are Conscious...................................23, 121

Esalen (Recordings)/Esalen (Stransky Notes)

E 2: Scanning - General Remarks
    Es 1: Scanning..19
E 23: Left Shoulder Differentiation and Reintegration Into the Self-Image
    Es 22: Left Shoulder, Lying on Side...100

E 24: Raising the Entire Self to Function With a Live Shoulder
  Es 23: Integrating Whole Body With the Improved Shoulder
  From Lesson 22...101
E 27: Primitive Locomotion: Coordinating the Locomotive Joints
  Es 25: Crawling on Knees...62, 96
E 35: Initiation in Rolling
  Es 33: Introduction to Rolling...95
E 46: Imagination and Action to Complete the Back-Self Image.............23

Alexander Yanai – Reels

1/2/2...54
10/2/4...92
10/4/3...96
12/2/1...108
12/3/5...109
13/1/1...80
13/1/2...52
16/1/1...78
16/1/2...54
17/1/1...64
17/1/2...64
17/2/1...64
19/2/4...65
19/2/5...65
19/4/3...88
2/2/2...109
2/3/2...109
2/3/5...108
2/4/1...3, 25
2/4/3...3, 25
20/2/1...89
21/1/3...15, 23, 26, 120

21/2/1...121
21/2/2...121
21/2/3...121
21/4/1...50, 82
22/2/2..73
22/3/2..94
22/3/3...53, 94
23/1/5..20, 121
23/2/1..21, 121
23/2/2..22
23/3/4..74
24/2/1..97
24/3/2...112
24/3/9..80
27/2/1...55, 95
27/2/4..75
3/4/4...75
31/3/3..89
32/3/2...107
33/1/1...67, 90
33/1/2...66, 90
33/1/3..91
33/1/4..92
33/3/3..59
33/3/4..60
33/4/1..59
34/3/2..63
35/4/2..51
4/1/4...111
4/2/4...111
4/4/2...61, 80
4/4/3..77

5/4/1..55
5/4/2..71
6/2/5..77
6/3/2..88
8/1/3..58
9/1/3...74, 121
9/1/6...74, 121
9/3/1..50
9/3/2..22
9/3/6..62

Collection of Twenty-Two Lessons

The twenty-two lessons in this collection have been selected as exemplary of the process of transformation described in this book. They include the construction of the body-self-image; the course of motor-sensorial development—from balancing to standing and walking; the renewal of habitual patterns; and the practice of body meditation, including scanning and imagination. The collection includes 19 individual Alexander Yanai (AY) lesson transcripts, and 3 audio recordings (MP3) of Moshe Feldenkrais's teaching at the Esalen Institute.

The International Feldenkrais Federation (IFF) offers the collection to accompany the book for instant download, here: https://feldenkrais-method.org/materials/item/the-power-of-self-transformation-the-feldenkrais-method/

AY 003 *Rolling to Sit With the Elbows*
AY 046 *Lowering the Head*
AY 057 *Lifting the Head on All Fours*
AY 058 *Transferring Support While on the Stomach*
AY 068 *Rolling the Fists*
AY 122 *Rolling Right and Left*
AY 145 *From Sitting to Standing While Turning*
AY 172 *Stopping the Breath*
AY 177 *Making the Spine Flexible and Integrating It*
AY 238 *Standing Backward, #2*
AY 275 *Introduction to Walking 2, continuation*
AY 313 *Rolling at the Rate of Stretching and Bending*
AY 327 *Sitting – Lying, continuation*
AY 338 *Primary Image*

AY 339 *Simpler*

AY 345 *Diagonal Image*

AY 417 *Preparation for Rolling to Sitting*

AY 502 *Walking and Crawling*

AY 513 *Reptiles*

E 2 *Scanning and General Remarks*

E 27 *Primitive Locomotion: Coordinating the Locomotive Joints*

E 46 *Imagination and Action to Complete the Back–Self Image*

Index of names and terms

acture, 49–50, 64, 66–67, 87, 90–91, 93
  see posture
arms, 12, 18, 20–22, 50, 52, 55, 57–58, 60, 66–67, 71–74, 76–77, 79–82, 87–92, 96–98, 100, 107, 109, 120
Asymmetrical tonic neck reflex (ATNR), 51, 71, 73– 75, 79
attunement, 37–38, 85
autosuggestion, 114–116
awareness, 5, 8, 15, 18–20, 22–24, 38, 46, 48, 52, 57, 66, 70, 74, 83, 85, 87, 99, 105–107, 109–110, 115, 119, 121, 127, 130, 132–133, 138
Awareness Through Movement (ATM), 2, 4, 23, 44, 120

balance, 5, 27, 49–50, 57–58, 65–66, 69, 72, 76–77, 79–81, 88–90, 92, 97, 105, 112
Baniel, 135
bipedalism, 28, 63–64, 91
body image, 8, 11, 14, 25, 35, 118
  see self-image
body meditation, 9, 105-106
  see meditation
bowing, 9, 106, 110–113
brain maps, 82, 135–137
brain plasticity, 34, 136
  see neuroplasticity
breathing, 5, 9, 19, 65, 70. 89, 106, 108–111, 117

cardinal lines, 18–19, 20, 22, 39, 106

chronic pain, 5, 32–33, 126
consciousness, 9, 12, 70, 85, 102, 105, 126–131, 139–140
Coué, Émile, 99–100, 115–117
crawling, 28, 30, 47–49, 56–63, 66, 69, 79–80, 87, 91, 96

Damasio, Antonio, 26, 31, 43, 83, 128–132, 139–140
Dead bird, 75, 86

eyes, 10, 19, 26, 75, 80, 86–87, 89, 96, 107

feelings, 6, 11, 13–14, 25–26, 28–29, 31, 34, 44, 46, 99–100, 113, 130
finger, 10, 20, 22, 24, 34, 81–82, 96, 107, 120,
Foucault, Michel, 138
Functional Integration (FI), 2, 35–39, 102, 135

Gallese, Vittorio, 118–119
gravity, 28, 49, 64, 67, 76–77, 79, 84, 111

habits, 16, 29, 84–86, 130, 139
head, 7, 15, 19, 20, 22, 32, 36, 46, 50, 52–54, 58–63, 65–67, 71–82, 86–87, 89–92, 94, 96–97, 100, 106, 109, 111–113, 118
heritage, 16, 69

hip, 20–22, 51–53, 56, 59–60, 62–63, 67, 72–74, 78, 90–91, 97–98, 100, 107, 119
homunculus, 26
imagination, 8, 23–24, 75, 105–106, 108, 117–121, 126

kinesthetic, 5, 8, 11, 38, 132
knees, 22, 50, 52, 55, 58–62, 65–66, 79–81, 86, 94, 96–97, 107, 109, 112–113

language, 16, 38, 44, 47, 133
legs, 18, 19–22, 51–53, 55, 58–63, 66, 73–77, 79–82, 88, 91, 94–95, 97, 100, 107
lengthening, 50–52, 73–74, 87

McGeoch, Paul, 34–35
meditation, 8, 105, 107, 113
　see body meditation
memory, 7–8, 26, 29, 31–33, 35, 57, 82, 126, 129, 131, 134
Merzenich, Michael, 136–137
midline, 52, 61, 72–73, 75, 79, 121
Moro reflex, 50, 81–82
motor development, 27, 30–31, 44–49, 52, 54–57, 61, 69, 76, 82, 87, 94, 127
mouth, 11, 52, 57, 70

neck, 7, 38, 53, 61, 63, 65–66, 79, 89, 101, 107
nervous system, 4, 6, 11–13, 16, 19, 27, 30, 33, 47, 57, 68, 70–71, 74, 84, 86, 100, 105, 130, 133
neuroplasticity, 9, 126, 133–135

neuroscience, 9, 26, 45, 118, 126, 128, 133–134, 136–137, 140
nonconscious, 9, 30, 33, 44, 45, 69, 84, 116–117, 121, 126–132

octopus, 12–13
ontogenetic, 27, 29

pain, 5, 28, 32, 34, 37, 46, 85, 116
　see chronic pain
phantom limb, 33–34, 126
posture, 5, 26, 28–29, 47–48, 50, 61, 64, 67, 69, 76–77, 79, 87, 88, 90–91, 93, 105, 110, 127, 130
　see acture
praying, 9, 34, 106, 111–113
Pribram, Karl, 38, 135
primitive reflexes, 30, 69, 74, 82, 117, 126, 130–131
　see reflexes
proprioception, 28, 49
psychoanalysis, 44
psychology, 25, 45, 126

reflexes, 8, 45, 47, 67–70, 82, 130
ribs, 7, 53, 655, 100, 109
Rizzolatti, Giacomo, 118
rolling, 21, 24, 28, 30, 46–49, 51–56, 61, 67, 71–72, 82, 92, 95–96, 121

scanning, 8–9, 19, 20, 22–24, 105–107, 117, 119, 134
Schilder, Paul, 25, 99–100
science, 32, 127

self-change, 2, 6–7, 17, 36, 46, 87, 105, 117–118, 126, 137–139

self-education, 16–18

self-healing, 5, 115

self-image, 6, 8, 11–24, 26, 28, 31, 36, 40, 46, 74, 83–84, 87, 102, 105–107, 117, 119, 127, 130, 133

self-transformation, 7–8, 18, 67, 84, 129, 130, 132

sensorial, 8–9, 15, 18, 24, 29, 31, 38, 49, 57, 69, 74, 101, 105, 115, 117, 120–121, 126, 130, 132

sensorimotor, 4, 6, 8, 15–17, 29–31, 35, 43–45, 47, 62, 67, 70, 84, 100, 126–127, 131

shoulder, 20–21, 51–52, 56, 58, 65, 67, 72, 74, 78, 88–91, 100–102, 109, 119

sitting, 4, 21, 28, 30, 46–49, 52–56, 60–62, 69, 72–73, 75, 84, 86–87, 94–97, 106, 109, 112

spine, 20–23, 28, 36, 52, 58, 61–63, 73–75, 77, 80, 97, 101, 106, 108, 110–112, 120

standing, 4, 7, 28, 30, 47–49, 51–52, 59–65, 69, 80, 82, 87–90, 94, 96–97, 112

Symmetrical tonic neck reflex (STNR), 8, 57, 61–62,, 74, 78–80

sucking, 70

sync, 6, 12, 15, 91

Tonic labyrinthine reflex (TLR), 74, 76–77, 79

transference, 90–100

transformation, 7–9, 43, 83–84, 100, 102, 118, 126, 129–132
    see self-transformation

unconscious, 45, 68, 70, 99, 103, 107, 109, 114, 16, 119, 127–129

walking, 4, 28, 36–37, 46–49, 55, 57–61, 82, 84, 87–92, 94, 97

Zemach-Bersin, David, 135

Selected Bibliography

Anālayo, Bhikkhu. 2020. "Buddhist Antecedents to the Body Scan Meditation." *Mindfulness* 11: 194–202.

Baniel, Anat. 2012. *Kids Beyond Limits: The Anat Baniel Method for Awakening the Brain and Transforming the Life of Your Child with Special Needs*. New York: Penguin Group.

Berne, Samuel A. 2006. "The Primitive Reflexes: Consideration in the Infant." *Optometry and Vision Development* 37 (3): 139–46.

Berthoz, Alain. 2000. *The Brain's Sense of Movement*. Translated by Giselle Weiss. Cambridge, MA: Harvard University Press.

Buckard, Christian. 2017. *Moshé Feldenkrais: Der Mensch hinter der Methode*. Munich, Germany: Piper.

Caruana, Fausto, and Italo Testa, eds. 2020. *Habits: Pragmatist Approaches from Cognitive Science, Neuroscience, and Social Theory*. New York: Cambridge University Press.

Ciofu, Anca-Mihaela. 2018. "The Feldenkrais Method in the Puppeteer's Training from the Perspective of Nicolas Gousseff's Handheld Puppets Workshops." *Review of Artistic Education* 15: 155–60.

Clark, Dav, Frank Schumann, and Stewart H. Mostofsky. 2015. "Mindful Movement and Skilled Attention." *Frontiers of Human Neuroscience* 9: 297. https://doi.org/10.3389 /fnhum.2015.00297.

Coué, Émile. 1922. *Self Mastery through Conscious Autosuggestion*. New York: Malkan Publishers.

Damasio, Antonio. 1999. *The Feeling of What Happens: Body and Emotion in the Making of Consciousness*. New York: Harcourt Brace.

------------ 2010. *Self Comes to Mind: Constructing the Conscious Brain*. New York: Pantheon Books.

------------- 2013. "Mental Self: The Person Within." *Nature* 423: 227.

Denk. Franziska, and Stephen B. McMahon. 2012. "Chronic Pain: Emerging Evidence for the Involvement of Epigenetics." *Neuron* 73: 435–44.

Doidge, Norman. 2007. *The Brain that Changes Itself*. New York: Viking Penguin.

------------- 2015. *The Brain's Way of Healing*. New York: Penguin.

Easton, Thomas A. 1972. "On the Normal Use of Reflexes." *American Scientist* 60 (5): 591–99.

Feldenkrais, Moshe. 1966. "Image, Movement, and Actor: Restoration and Potentiality." *The Tulane Drama Review* 10 (3): 112–26.

------------- 1980. *Feldenkrais Professional Training Program Transcript*. Amherst, Massachusetts. Week One. Edited by Bonnie R. Humiston, 2007

------------- 1981. Quest Seminar: New York, 1981. Discussion: "Habits. Fear: We are not interested in moving but in how the movement is performed." Audio set. San Diego, CA: Feldenkrais Resources.

------------- 1981. *The Elusive Obvious or Basic Feldenkrais*. Capitola, CA: Meta Publications.

------------- 1984. *The Master Moves*. Capitola, CA: Meta Publications.

------------- 1985. *The Potent Self: A Study of Spontaneity and Compulsion*. Berkeley, CA: Frog Books.

------------- 2005 [1949]. *Body and Mature Behavior: A Study of Anxiety, Sex, Gravitation, and Learning*. Berkeley, CA: Somatic Resources/Frog Books.

------------- 2006. *San Francisco Evening Class Notes, 1976*. Edited by Richard Ehrman. Revised edition. San Diego, CA: Feldenkrais Resources.

------------ 2009 [1972]. *Awareness Through Movement: Easy-to-Do Health Exercises to Improve Your Posture, Vision, Imagination, and Personal Awareness*. San Francisco: Harper One.

------------ 2010. *Embodied Wisdom: The Collected Papers of Moshe Feldenkrais*. Edited by Elizabeth Beringer. Berkeley, CA: Somatic Resources and North Atlantic Books.

------------ 2012. *Esalen 1972 Workshop: Judith Stransky Notes*. San Diego, CA: Feldenkrais Resources.

------------ 2013 [1929]. *Thinking and Doing: A Monograph by Moshe Feldenkrais*. Longmont, CO: Genesis II Publishing.

------------ 2013. *1974 London ATM Workshop*. Feldenkrais Resources: San Diego, CA.

Feldenkrais, Moshe, and Pribram, Karl. 2006. Tape: "The Feldenkrais–Pribram Discussions—San Francisco 1975." Paris, France: International Feldenkrais Federation.

Feldy Notebook. https://feldynotebook.com/.

Foucault, Michel. 1988a. *The Care of the Self*. Vol. 3 in *The History of Sexuality*. Translated by Robert Hurley. New York: Vintage Books.

------------ 1988b. "The Ethic of Care for the Self as a Practice of Freedom: An Interview with Michel Foucault." In *The Final Foucault*, edited by James Bernauer and David Rasmussen, 1–20. Cambridge, MA: The MIT Press.

------------ 2005. *The Hermeneutics of the Subject: Lectures at the Collège de France, 1981–82*. Translated by Graham Burchell. New York: Palgrave Macmillan.

Fredricksson, E. Krystin. 2017. *Awareness Through Puppetry: Self-Image in Feldenkrais Method and Material Performance*. Ph.D. Thesis. Royal Holloway, University of London, Department of Drama and Theatre Studies.

Gallese, Vittorio, Luciano Fadiga, Leonardo Fogassi, and Giacomo Rizzolatti. 1996. "Action Recognition in the Premotor Cortex." *Brain* 119: 593–609.

Godfrey-Smith, Peter. 2017. *Other Minds: The Octopus, the Sea, and the Deep Origins of Consciousness.* London and Glasgow, UK: William Collins.

Graybiel, M. Ann. 2008. "Habits, Rituals, and the Evaluative Brain." *Annual Review of Neuroscience* 31: 359–87.

Grogan, Sarah. 2007. *Body Image: Understanding Body Dissatisfaction in Men, Women and Children.* London: Routledge.

Hancock, Dianne. 2015. "Teaching the Feldenkrais Method in UK Higher Education Performer Training." *Theatre, Dance and Performance Training* 6 (2): 59–173.

Henderson, Hester L., Ron French, and Paul McCarty. 1993. "ATNR: It's [sic] Possible Impact on the Motor Efficiency of Children." *The Physical Educator* 50 (1): 20–26.

Higgins, Susan. 1991. "Motor Skill Acquisition." *Physical Therapy* 71 (2): 123–39.

Hillier, Susan, and Anthea Worley. 2015. "The Effectiveness of the Feldenkrais Method: A Systematic Review of the Evidence." *Evidence-Based Complementary and Alternative Medicine* 2015.

Ianì, Francesco. 2019. "Embodied memories: Reviewing the role of the body in memory processes." *Psychonomic Bulletin and Review* 26: 1747–66.

Kamm, Kathi, Esther Thelen, and Jody L. Jensen. 1990. "A Dynamical Systems Approach to Motor Development." *Physical Therapy* 70 (12): 763–75.

Kilteni, Konstantina, Benjamin Jan Andersson, Christian Houborg, and H. Henrik Ehrsson. 2018. "Motor Imagery Involves Predicting the Sensory Consequences of Imagined Movement." *Nature Communications* 9 (1): 1617.

Le Huec, Jean Charles, R. Saddiki, Jörg Franke, J. Rigal, and Stéphane Aunoble. 2011. "Equilibrium of the Human Body and the Gravity Line: The Basics." *European Spine Journal* 20 (5): 558–63.

Mansbach, Abraham. 2016. "Becoming Ourselves: Feldenkrais and Foucault on Soma and Culture." *Feldenkrais Research Journal,* vol. 5. https://feldenkraisresearchjournal.org.

McGeoch, Paul, and Vilayanur S. Ramachandran. 2012. "The Appearance of New Phantom Fingers Post-Amputation in a Phocomelus." *Neurocase* 18 (2): 95–97.

Melzack, Ronald, and Patrick D. Wall, eds. 2003. *Handbook of Pain Management.* London: Churchill Livingston.

Mental Health Foundation. 2019. "Body Image: How We Think and Feel about Our Bodies." London: Mental Health Foundation, https://www.mentalhealth.org.uk/publications/body-image-report.

Merzenich, Michael. 2012. "Dr. Michael Merzenich on Neuroscience, Learning and the Feldenkrais Method; in conversation with Cliff Smyth." The Feldenkrais Guild of North America, https://www.youtube.com/ watch?v=rupZ-wlRdA0. Accessed 13 September 2021.

-------------- 2013. *Soft-Wired: How the New Science of Brain Plasticity can Change Your Life.* San Francisco CA: Parnassus Publishing.

Payne, V. Gregory, and Larry D. Isaacs. 2016. *Human Motor Development: A Lifespan Approach.* New York, N.Y: Routledge.

Porges, Stephen W. 2011. *The Polyvagal Theory: Neurophysiological Foundations of Emotions, Attachment, Communication, and Self-Regulation.* New York: W. W. Norton.

Reese, Mark. 2015. *Moshe Feldenkrais: A Life in Movement*. San Rafael, CA: ReeseKress Somatics Press.

Rizzolatti, Giacomo, and Michael A. Arbib. 1998. "Language within Our Grasp." *Trends in Neurosciences* 21 (5): 188–94.

Rizzolatti, Giacomo. 2005. "The Mirror Neuron System and Its Function in Humans." *Anatomy and Embryology* (Berlin) 210 (5–6): 419–21.

Schilder, Paul Ferdinand. 1935. *The Image and Appearance of the Human Body*. London: Kegan Paul.

Shelhav, Chava. 2019. *Child Space: An Integrated Approach to Infant Development Based on the Feldenkrais Method*. Berkeley, CA: North Atlantic Books and Somatic Resources.

Sholl, Robert, ed. 2021. *The Feldenkrais Method in Creative Practice: Dance, Music and Theatre*. London: Bloomsbury.

Speransky, Alekseĭ D. 1943. *A Basis for the Theory of Medicine*. Translated by C. P. Dutt. New York: International Publishers.

Turner, Bryan S., ed. 2012. *The Routledge Handbook of Body Studies*. New York: Routledge.

Wagner, Nils-Frederic, and Georg Northoff. 2014. "Habits: Bridging the Gap between Personhood and Personal Identity." *Frontiers in Human Neuroscience* 8: 330. https://doi.org/10.3389/fnhum.2014.00330

Yeatman, Anna. 2007. "Freedom and the Feldenkrais Method." *Feldenkrais Research Journal* 3. http://iffresearchjournal.org/ volume/3/yeatman.

Zemach-Bersin, David. 2012. Introduction to *Esalen 1972 Workshop: Judith Stransky Notes*. San Diego, CA: Feldenkrais Resources.